OPIOID EDUCATION

ALTERNATIVE

TREATMENTS

FOR PAIN MANAGEMENT

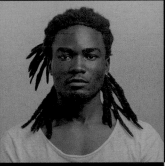

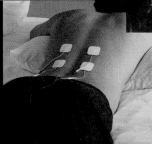

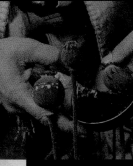

PAINKILLERS: THE SCOURGE ON SOCIETY

ALTERNATIVE TREATMENTS FOR PAIN MANAGEMENT

HOW FIRST RESPONDERS AND ER DOCTORS SAVE LIVES AND EDUCATE

TREATMENTS FOR OPIOID ADDICTION

UNDERSTANDING DRUG USE AND ADDICTION

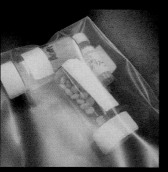

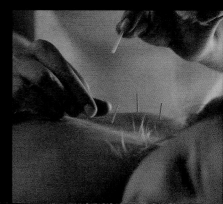

OPIOID EDUCATION

ALTERNATIVE
TREATMENTS
FOR PAIN MANAGEMENT

BEN BAKER

MASON CREST
PHILADELPHIA | MIAMI

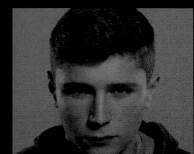

MASON CREST
450 Parkway Drive, Suite D, Broomall, Pennsylvania 19008
(866) MCP-BOOK (toll-free) • www.masoncrest.com

© 2020 by Mason Crest, an imprint of National Highlights, Inc.

Printed and bound in the United States of America.

CPSIA Compliance Information: Batch #OE2019.
For further information, contact Mason Crest at 1-866-MCP-Book.

First printing

ISBN (hardback) 978-1-4222-4382-4
ISBN (series) 978-1-4222-4378-7
ISBN (ebook) 978-1-4222-7429-3

Library of Congress Cataloging-in-Publication Data on file at the Library of Congress

Interior and cover design: Torque Advertising + Design
Interior layout: Tara Raymo, CreativelyTara
Production: Michelle Luke

Publisher's Note: Websites listed in this book were active at the time of publication. The publisher is not responsible for websites that have changed their address or discontinued operation since the date of publication. The publisher reviews and updates the websites each time the book is reprinted.

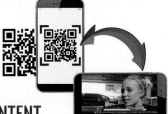

QR CODES AND LINKS TO THIRD-PARTY CONTENT

CONTENTS

KEY ICONS TO LOOK FOR:

 Words to Understand: These words with their easy-to-understand definitions will increase the reader's understanding of the text while building vocabulary skills.

 Sidebars: This boxed material within the main text allows readers to build knowledge, gain insights, explore possibilities, and broaden their perspectives by weaving together additional information to provide realistic and holistic perspectives.

 Educational videos: Readers can view videos by scanning our QR codes, providing them with additional educational content to supplement the text. Examples include news coverage, moments in history, speeches, iconic sports moments, and much more!

 Text-Dependent Questions: These questions send the reader back to the text for more careful attention to the evidence presented there.

 Research Projects: Readers are pointed toward areas of further inquiry connected to each chapter. Suggestions are provided for projects that encourage deeper research and analysis.

 Series Glossary of Key Terms: This back-of-the-book glossary contains terminology used throughout this series. Words found here increase the reader's ability to read and comprehend higher-level books and articles in this field.

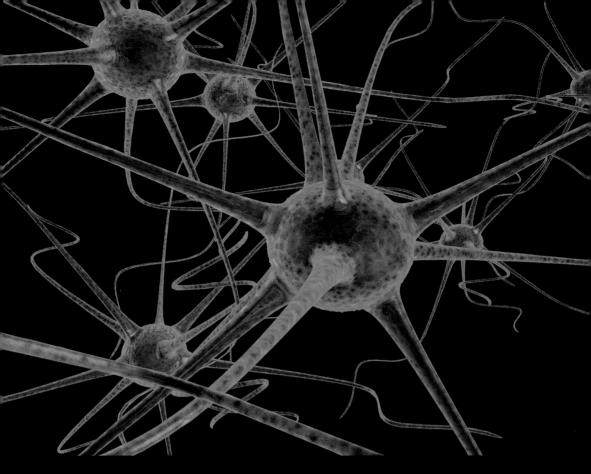

Feelings of pain are communicated through the central nervous system. These pain messages warn the brain when the body is being damaged.

 WORDS TO UNDERSTAND

congenital—a physical characteristic that is inherited genetically from one or both parents.

limbic system—the nerves and network in the brain that controls instincts and mood. It controls basic emotions like fear, happiness and anger and urges like hunger.

nociception—the process through which nerves transmit pain sensations to the brain, from the Latin word for "hurt."

CHAPTER 1

WHAT IS PAIN?

What is pain? It is easy to answer "something that hurts," but that does not explain what pain really is. Everyone feels pain when they are hurt, but each person experiences pain in different ways. The International Association for the Study of Pain defines pain as "the unpleasant sensory and emotional experience associated with actual or potential tissue damage, or described in terms of such damage."

Medical writer Adam Felman goes a little further in trying to explain the purpose of pain. "Pain is an unpleasant sensation and emotional experience linked to tissue damage. Its purpose is to allow the body to react and prevent further tissue damage," he wrote in *Medical News Today*. "We feel pain when a signal is sent through nerve fibers to the brain for interpretation. The experience of pain is different for everyone, and there are different ways of feeling and describing pain. This can make it difficult to define and treat.

Peripheral Nervous System

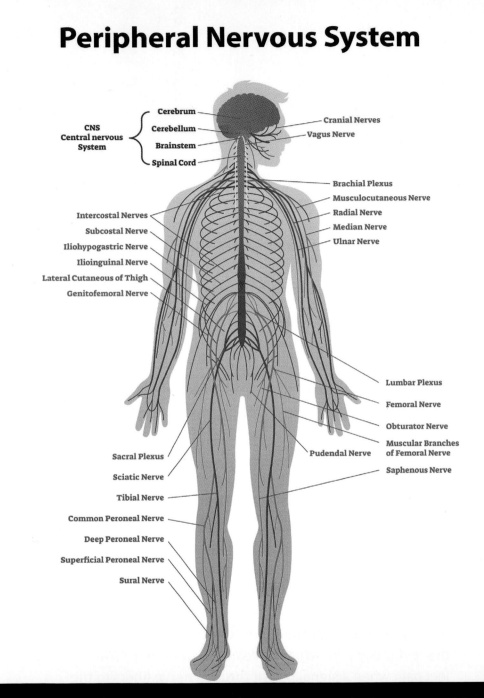

CNS
Central nervous
System

- Cerebrum
- Cerebellum
- Brainstem
- Spinal Cord

- Cranial Nerves
- Vagus Nerve

- Brachial Plexus
- Musculocutaneous Nerve
- Radial Nerve
- Median Nerve
- Ulnar Nerve

Intercostal Nerves
Subcostal Nerve
Iliohypogastric Nerve
Ilioinguinal Nerve
Lateral Cutaneous of Thigh
Genitofemoral Nerve

Lumbar Plexus
Femoral Nerve
Obturator Nerve
Muscular Branches
of Femoral Nerve

Pudendal Nerve

Sacral Plexus
Sciatic Nerve

Saphenous Nerve

Tibial Nerve
Common Peroneal Nerve
Deep Peroneal Nerve
Superficial Peroneal Nerve
Sural Nerve

The peripheral nervous system includes the network of nerves outside the central nervous system. These nerves, which run through the body, communicate pain and other sensations to the brain.

Pain can be short-term or long-term, it can stay in one place, or it can spread around the body."

How Pain Works

The body uses pain to communicate to the brain that something is wrong. For example, consider what happens when a person inadvertently puts her hand on a hot stove burner. The heat immediately begins to damage skin tissue. This activates microscopic pain receptors in the skin, which are located at one end of a nerve cell. The activated receptors send a pain message that says "something is wrong" to the other end of the nerve cell, which is connected to the body's central nervous system in the spinal cord.

After the pain message, which is in the form of an electrical signal, reaches the spinal cord, the message continues to move toward the brain. The pain message signal is transmitted by means of special chemicals, called neurotransmitters, which are released by the nerve cells. These help the message to cross over the gaps (synapses) between nerve cells.

The transmission of pain signals happens very quickly, but the body reacts to pain even before the brain recognizes what is happening. When pain receptors are activated, the central nervous system instantly generates a reflex response. For the person who accidentally touched the hot stove, the reflex response would be for her arm muscles to contract, jerking her hand away from the source of the tissue damage. This happens involuntarily, before the brain has even received and processed the pain message.

Once the pain message reaches the brain, it goes to an area called the thalamus. This part of the brain sorts through all different types of signals, and sends them to an area of the brain that can act on them. Pain messages are sent to three areas: the somatosensory cortex, which is responsible for physical sensation; the frontal cortex, which is in charge of thinking; and the **limbic system**, which is linked to emotions. These three areas all react to pain. The person who

 ## THE NERVOUS SYSTEM

The nervous system is the body's collection of nerves. A nerve is a little like an electrical wire. It transmits signals from the body to the brain and back.

The nervous system starts with the brain and runs through the spinal cord. From there, nerves branch out through the rest of the body. Interestingly enough, the brain itself cannot feel pain. People who have brain surgery have their nerves deadened with medicine so they won't feel painful incisions in their scalp or bone, but the brain itself does not need such treatment.

The peripheral nerve systems outside the brain and spinal column can be broken into two groups. The somatic nervous system transmits sensations, such as hot, cold, hard, soft, and more. This is where pain is generated. The autonomic nervous system controls muscle movement. Autonomic nerves control breathing, blinking, heartbeats, and other body actions like lifting an arm or moving eyes back and forth to read these words. The autonomic system causes a hand to jerk away from something that is burning hot.

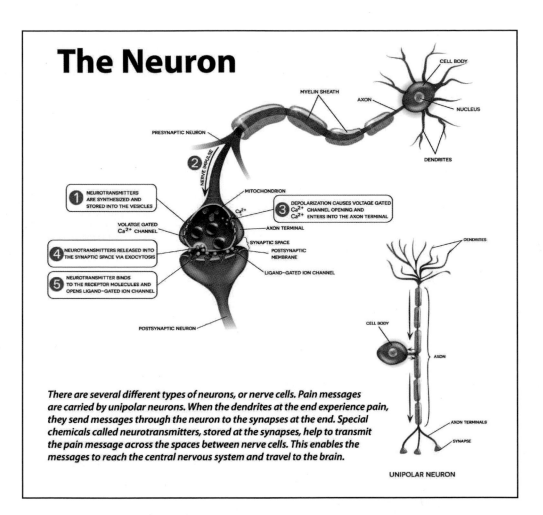

The Neuron

There are several different types of neurons, or nerve cells. Pain messages are carried by unipolar neurons. When the dendrites at the end experience pain, they send messages through the neuron to the synapses at the end. Special chemicals called neurotransmitters, stored at the synapses, help to transmit the pain message across the spaces between nerve cells. This enables the messages to reach the central nervous system and travel to the brain.

has touched the hot stove notices the unpleasant physical sensation, thinks, "Ow, that hurts!" and feels irritated, upset, or annoyed. This transmission of pain signals is called **nociception**, from the Latin word for "hurt."

Acute and Chronic Pain

When people experience physical pain, they may decide to seek medical care. The health care professional attending to them performs a physical examination and run some tests to determine where the issue lies. Once they understand

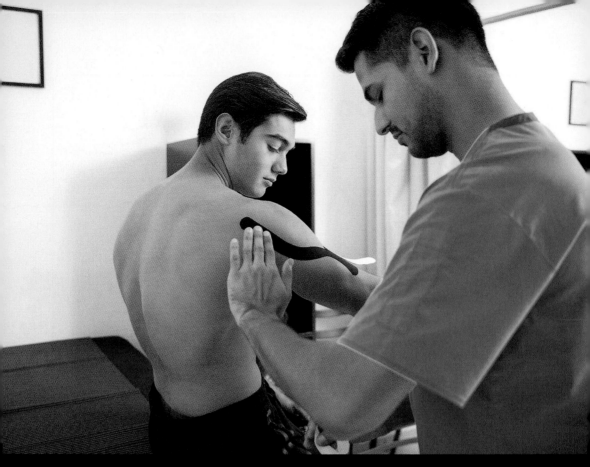

Acute pain is usually caused by physical injuries. This type of pain typically disappears within a few weeks or months when appropriate treatment is given. But acute pain can turn into chronic pain if the cause of the underlying pain remains untreated.

why the patient is in pain, some form of treatment—such as medication or physical therapy—is prescribed. If all goes well, the patient begins to heal, and eventually they are able to return to their daily life.

In most cases, the pain that accompanies an injury is acute pain. This is short-lived pain that tells the body that damage is occurring, or has occurred. Acute pain can be treated at the same time that the injury is treated. As the injury heals, the acute pain also recedes.

Scan here to learn more about chronic pain:

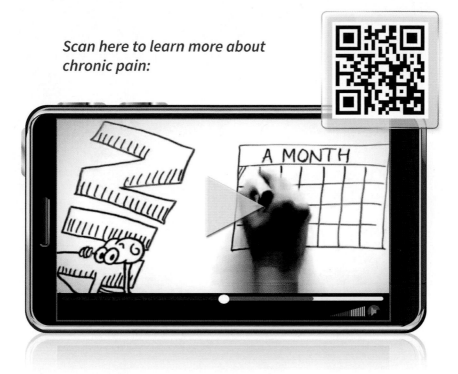

Some patients never fully heal, or suffer from long-term health conditions or diseases that force them to live with pain for months or years. Chronic pain is defined as pain that lasts for at least three to six consecutive months, or is present for three to six months nonconsecutively during a twelve-month period. It can be caused by inflammations of tissue (for example, arthritis), or by damage to nerves caused by diseases like diabetes or shingles. Sometimes, the cause of chronic pain can't be determined.

People Experience Pain Differently

Pain is different for everyone because everyone has a different pain threshold. A pain threshold is how much a pain a person can stand. In addition, the ways in which the body reacted to

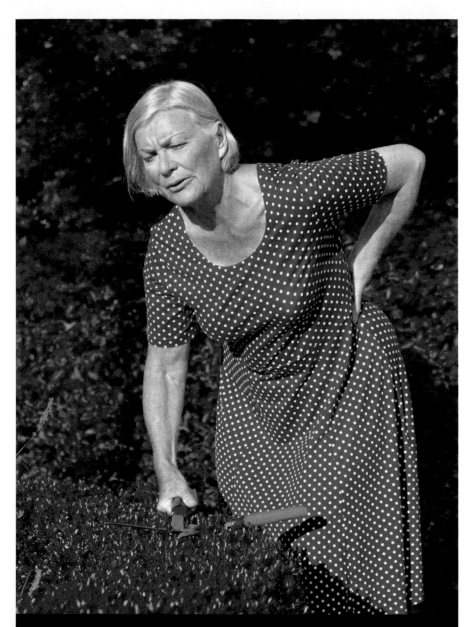

In 2018, the Centers for Disease Control estimated that 50 million Americans—more than 20 percent of the adult population—suffer from chronic pain. About 20 million of them suffer from "high-impact chronic pain"—pain that is severe enough to frequently limit their lifestyle or work activities.

a painful situation in the past can affect how it reacts to the same kind of pain the next time it occurs.

Pain thresholds can vary in a person over time. As people age, their brain loses cells. This reduces the amount of pain an older person can handle. As a result, elderly people often have more problems with pain than younger people. Even a person's gender can affect how they experience pain. "Research shows that women have a higher sensitivity to pain than men do," writes Craig Freudenrich. "This could be because of sex-linked genetic traits and hormonal changes that might alter the pain perception system."

Brain damage can also affect how the body reacts to pain. When someone has a stroke, a blood clot cuts off the blood supply to part of the brain. That part of the brain dies, and the person loses some brain function, at least temporarily. If the damage was to a small part of the brain, the rest of the brain can eventually take over the missing abilities and responsibilities. This takeover is not perfect, however. The National Stroke Association says a stroke can leave a person with long-term pain:

> Central post-stroke pain is described as constant, moderate, or severe pain caused by damage to the brain. This means that after a stroke, your brain does not understand normal messages sent from the body in response to touch, warmth, cold, and other stimuli. Instead, the brain may register even slight sensations on your skin as painful.

When a person is overly tired, pain is felt more. Lack of sleep stresses the brain. The brain responds by boosting the reaction to pain signals. In this case, the brain is saying it needs time to rest and recuperate.

Measuring Pain

When a person visits the doctor's office complaining of pain, a doctor or nurse may ask them to identify how much it hurts on a pain scale. This is a tool that can be used to measure the severity, duration, or type of pain. The patient usually self-reports where their pain falls on a specially designed range: zero might be no pain, two might be mild pain, five might be moderate pain, and ten would be the worst pain imaginable. Pain scales exist for people of all ages, from young children to senior citizens.

Doctors use pain scales to better understand certain aspects of their patients' pain. The scales can help them make accurate diagnoses, create treatment plans, and measure the effectiveness of treatment.

A problem with pain scales is that all people feel pain differently. During the 1940s, researchers at the University of Cornell tried to create a scale for pain that could apply to everyone. The scale was called a "dol." The scientists took

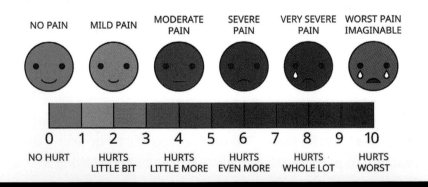

PAIN MEASUREMENT SCALE

Pain measurement scales like this one help young people to tell doctors about the level of discomfort they are feeling.

Some people have tried to manage pain in non-medicinal ways. Meditating is a way that some people take their mind off of problems that they are dealing with. By focusing on something other than pain, the meditator attempts to control the pain. Physical massages can loosen tense muscles and relieve pain by promoting better blood flow. And eating certain types of healthy foods can naturally reduce pain. For example, olive oil reduces inflammation, a leading cause of pain, and is good for heart health. Foods that are high in Omega-3 fatty acids, such as fish and nuts, or antioxident-rich foods like blueberries and cherries, can also help to reduce inflammation.

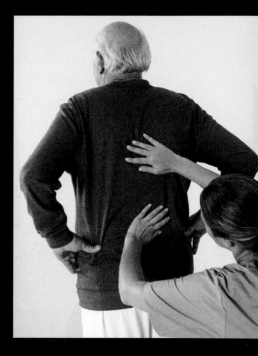

women who were in the process of having children ("in labor") and burned their hands. (The women had volunteered for this study.) The problem was that some women were more tolerant to the burning than others. One lady's skin blistered and charred from third-degree burns before she said it was too much. Ultimately, the "dol" scale was never adopted.

There are a tiny number of people who do not feel pain at all. This is due to an inherited genetic condition called

congenital insensitivity. The condition is dangerous: pain is a warning to the body that something is wrong. A person with this condition could be critically burned in a fire and not even realize it until it is too late.

Very few people in the world—maybe fewer than 7,500 people total—have this congenital insensitivity. Ashlyn Blocker, a resident of the state of Georgia, is one of them. If a knife were pushed against her skin, she says, she would feel pressure, but not pain. Another person with this condition is Steven Pete, of Washington state. He once broke his back in three places—but didn't realize it for eight months. "There's no way I could live a normal life right now if I could actually feel pain," he told an interviewer, explaining that he would probably be constrained to a bed or wheelchair from all the damage his body has sustained over the years. Scientific researchers are studying people like Ashlyn and Steven, in hopes of learning more about how the body processes pain, in order to develop new treatments for chronic pain.

TEXT-DEPENDENT QUESTIONS

1. What is pain and how is it experienced?
2. What three areas of the brain receive pain messages?
3. What is the difference between acute and chronic pain?

RESEARCH PROJECT

Is pain and pain management a problem in your community? Talk to doctors or medical providers about the kinds of pain they see in patients. If you know older people who take pain medication, ask them how they feel about their medicine. Ask what they know about non-prescription pain management. How does chronic pain affect the way they live. Write a one-page essay about how pain affects people.

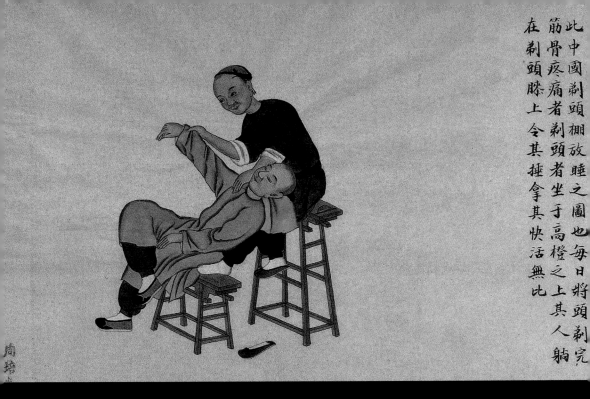

在剃頭膝上令其捶拿其快活無比

筋骨疼痛者剃頭者坐于高櫈之上其人躺

此中國剃頭棚放睡之圖也每日將頭剃完

A Chinese print from the late nineteenth century shows a man being treated for pain in his shoulder. Techniques and drugs for pain relief have been sought since ancient times.

WORDS TO UNDERSTAND

anesthetic—a drug that makes a person insensitive to pain, often used for surgery.

epidemic—a widespread health problem, usually one with the potential to be fatal. The opioid addiction crisis is an epidemic in some communities because it affects so many people.

opioid—term for a group of substances that activate certain receptors in the human brain, proving pleasure and painkilling effects.

trepanning—cutting a hole in the skull of a living person, which was done by ancient healers in order to release evils spirits thought to be trapped in a sick person's body.

CHAPTER 2

PAIN TREATMENT THROUGH HISTORY

Throughout recorded human history, people have tried to reduce or eliminate pain. In the most primitive communities, painkilling efforts may have involved healers shaking rattles or performing sacrifices or rituals that were believed to help sick people get better.

As ancient civilizations developed, medicine evolved. The ancient Egyptians extracted oil from myrrh trees and used it for healing. In China and the Indus River Valley, extensive traditions of herbal medicine evolved thousands of years ago. Chinese and Indian healers employed a variety of plants (such as ginseng root, ginkgo biloba, and cinnamon), animal parts (rinocerous horn and snake oil) and even some mineral substances that are toxic to the human body in larger amounts (arsenic, lead, and mercury). An important Chinese reference text is the *Great Compendium of Herbs*, written by a Chinese doctor in the sixteenth century, Li Shizhen. The Indian system of traditional medicine is known as Ayurveda.

All over the world, natural substances were used to ease pain. Some of these substances are still used today in one form or another. For example, nearly 6,000 years ago, the ancient Sumerians discovered that sap from the opium poppy (*papaver somniferum*) could be used to reduce pain and help people relax. Opium was used as a painkilling medicine in the Roman Empire, and later in Renaissance Europe, as well

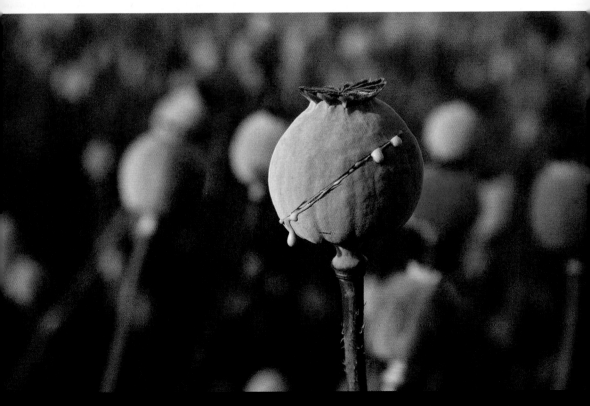

*The whitish sap of the opium poppy (*papaver somniferum*) can be processed into opium, morphine, heroin, and codeine—a group of drugs known as opiates. These drugs are very effective painkillers but also highly addictive.*

as throughout Asia. During the nineteenth century, German scientists processed raw opium into the powerful painkilling drugs morphine and heroin. Morphine is still used today, as are synthetic drugs called **opioids** that have the same painkilling effect on the brain as opium, morphine, and heroin. These drugs are effective but can be highly addictive when misused.

In the Andean highlands of South America, natives chewed on the leaves of the coca plant to numb pain and gain an energy boost. Coca leaves can be processed into cocaine. Although this drug is illegal to use recreationally, it is considered by the US government to have a legitimate medical use as a pain-reducing **anesthetic** for certain types of surgery.

Since ancient times, indigenous people from all over the world chewed the bark of willow trees to fight painful fevers and inflammations. Willow tree bark includes the chemical compound acetylsalicylic acid—which today is sold as the painkilling drug aspirin.

Alcohol, known for its intoxicating effects, is another of the oldest pain treatments. Alcohol occurs naturally wherever sugars ferment so it is found throughout the world. "People have used alcohol to relieve pain since ancient times," notes the National Institute of Alcohol Abuse and Alcoholism. "Laboratory studies confirm that alcohol does indeed reduce pain in humans and in animals. Moreover, recent research suggests that as many as 28 percent of people experiencing chronic pain turn to alcohol to alleviate their suffering. Despite this, using alcohol to alleviate pain places people at risk for a number of harmful health consequences."

Natural drugs were often used in primitive medical procedures. For example, there is evidence that more than 3,500 years ago indigenous people in the Andean highlands of South America occasionally performed a surgical procedure called **trepanning**. This involved drilling a hole in the skull of a living person. The superstitious natives believed this would "release evil spirits," but the procedure may have had an inadvertent medical benefit by relieving pressure caused by head injuries. The practice was still in use when Spanish conquistadores arrived in Inca Empire of Peru. They described Peruvian healers chewing coca leaves into a paste, which was spit into the wound to spread this plant's numbing effects. The discovery of skulls that show new bone growth around the holes indicate that patients did survive this crude procedure.

The Development of Modern Opioids

During the Renaissance period in Europe, a substance called laudanum was the most popular medicine for pain. The original form was developed by a Swiss doctor and alchemist named Paracelsus in the sixteenth century. Paracelsus's laudanum included a small amount of opium, as well as other ingredients such as citrus juice and powdered gold. Over the next three centuries, a variety of other laudanum formulas would be sold, including some that included alcohol. One of the most popular was produced by an English physician named Thomas Sydenham in the 1680s, which became popular across Europe. Laudanum was widely used to treat everything from pain and insomnia to various diseases. It was even used to quiet crying babies.

In the late eighteenth century and the early nineteenth century, many scientists were trying to understand how opium caused its painkilling effects. In 1803, a German chemist named Freidrich Serturner isolated the active ingredient in opium, which he named morphine. (The name is derived from Morpheus, the Greek god of sleep.)

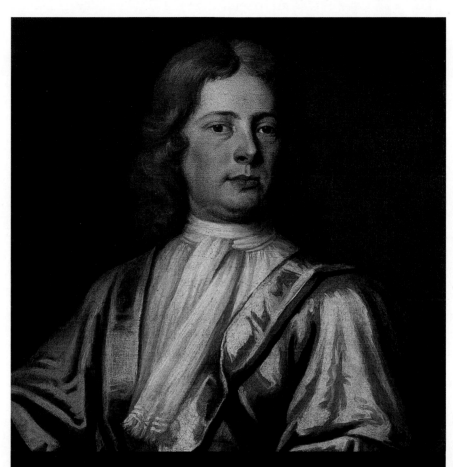

The English physician Thomas Sydenham (1624–1689) is sometimes called the "father of English medicine." His formula for laudanum was a popular cure for various ailments during the seventeenth and eighteenth centuries.

After the invention of the hypodermic needle in the 1850s, morphine was used for chronic pain, in surgical procedures, and in combination with other general sedatives. But, like opium, morphine had a high potential for abuse, and was not very safe to use. As a result, pain researchers spent a lot of time trying to develop a safer, more effective, non-addicting opiate.

In the United States, drugs are placed into five categories, known as schedules, to help identify risk of abuse and dependency as well as the appropriate medical uses, if any, for the drug. Schedule I drugs such as ecstasy, heroin, and LSD are among the most dangerous drugs. These drugs have a high potential for abuse and have no legitimate medical uses. Schedule II drugs include cocaine, as well as opiates like oxycodone, fentanyl, and methadone. They have legitimate medical uses, but all carry a high potential for abuse and can cause serious physical or psychological dependence.

Schedule III drugs include ketamine and Tylenol-Codeine, which have a moderate to low potential for physical and psychological dependence. Schedule IV drugs, such as Tramadol, Xanax, Valium, and Ambien, have a low potential for abuse and dependency. Schedule V drugs, such as cough syrups with under 200 milligrams of codeine, contain limited amounts of specific narcotics and have the lowest potential for abuse.

The drug schedules were created by a federal law, the Controlled Substances Act of 1970. Two government agencies, the Drug Enforcement Administration (DEA) and the Food and Drug Administration (FDA), determine which substances are added to or removed from the official drug schedules.

In the late nineteenth century, a new drug called diacetylmorphine was synthesized from morphine by scientists working for the Bayer pharmaceutical company in Elberfeld, Germany. Bayer gave this new drug the name Heroin, and introduced it to the world in 1895. The name was probably derived from *heroisch*, German medical terminology for "powerful," "large," or "extreme." Bayer promoted Heroin as the answer for many medical problems. It was used in pain-relieving syrups, as well as cold and cough medicines.

Bayer promoted Heroin as a safer, non-addictive alternative to morphine. However, within a few years doctors and scientists began to realize that the drug was actually *more* addictive than morphine. In the early 1900s Bayer removed the drug from the market.

During the twentieth century, new drugs were created in laboratories and intended to mimic the effects of the opium-based drugs (opiates). These drugs were not directly derived

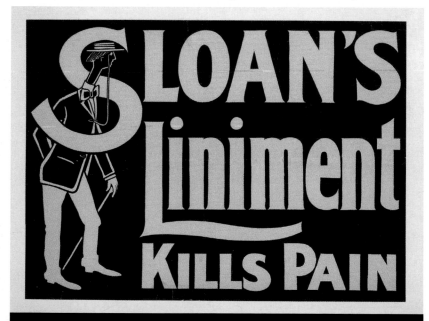

Advertisement for Sloan's Liniment, a nineteenth-century cream promoted for relieving muscle aches and joint pain. The product, which is still available today, utilized capsaicin, the active ingredient in chili peppers that makes them hot.

from the opium poppy, so they were called opioids. Among the first were oxycodone, which was synthesized in 1917, and hydromorphone, which was first produced in 1922. Later opioids included Fentanyl, synthesized in 1949. All of these were effective painkillers. But due to their high potential for abuse, addiction, and overdose, opioids in general were usually prescribed only to cancer patients and people experiencing excruciating, acute pain.

Increasing Use of Opioids

During the early 1990s, opioid pills that gradually released the drug into the patients' system were developed. They were called "extended release" or "long release" pills, which made them more effective for treating chronic pain. One of these drugs was an extended release version of oxycodone sold under the brand name OxyContin.

OxyContin was originally prescribed to relieve serious pain associated with cancer. But in 1996 the drug's manufacturer, Purdue Pharma, began encouraging doctors to prescribe OxyContin and other opioids to treat all types of pain, including toothaches and back pain. In educational programs for doctors, and in literature promoting their products, Purdue and other drug companies greatly downplayed their medications' potential for addiction while exaggerating their effectiveness. As a result, physicians had the impression that prescription painkillers were much safer and more effective for chronic pain than they truly were. Between 1996 and 2011, opioid pain reliever use in the United States doubled and oxycodone use grew almost fivefold.

Independent researchers found little evidence to support the claims that Purdue Pharma and other pharmaceutical companies were making about the benefits and safety of

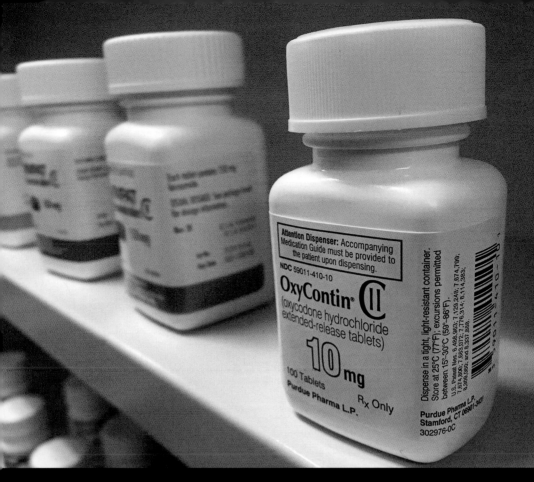

OxyContin is a popular brand of opioid painkiller in which the drug is slowly released into the person's system over a twelve-hour period. It comes in various strengths, from 10 to 80 milligrams.

opioid painkillers. Instead, they discovered overwhelming evidence pointing to the potential for abuse, addiction, overdose, falls, fractures, constipation, sexual dysfunction, and heart attacks.

In 2007, executives from Purdue Pharma acknowledged in federal court that the company had made misleading statements to doctors about OxyContin's effectiveness and safety. Purdue Pharma was fined $600 million, but by this point it was too late. An opioid problem had begun in the United States.

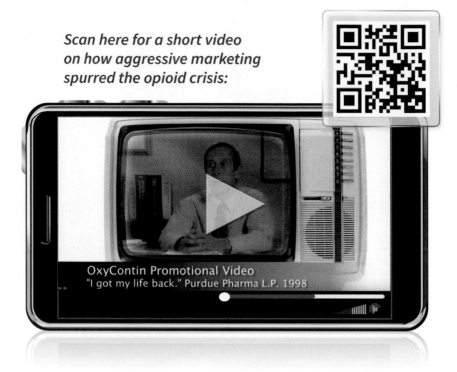

Scan here for a short video on how aggressive marketing spurred the opioid crisis:

OxyContin Promotional Video
"I got my life back." Purdue Pharma L.P. 1998

Today, that problem has grown into a full-blown crisis. Since 1999, the rate of drug overdose deaths in the United States has skyrocketed. Opioid drugs have largely driven the increase: in 2018 over 70,000 deaths occurred because of opioid overdoses, and more than half of them involved prescription painkillers.

"Every day, more than 130 people in the United States die after overdosing on opioids," notes the National Institute on Drug Abuse. "The misuse of and addiction to opioids—including prescription pain relievers, heroin, and synthetic opioids such as fentanyl—is a serious national crisis that affects public health as well as social and economic welfare."

Unfortunately, the opioid **epidemic** has been perpetuated by doctors and pharmacists. Some pharmacists are merely

DRUG OVERDOSE DEATHS IN THE UNITED STATES, 1999-2017

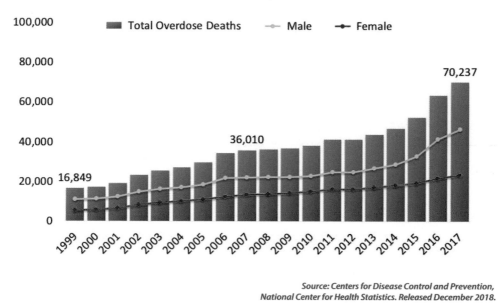

Source: Centers for Disease Control and Prevention, National Center for Health Statistics. Released December 2018.

The rate of drug overdose deaths increased from 6.1 per 100,000 people in 1999 to 21.7 in 2017. The rate rose by 10 percent a year from 1999 through 2006, by 3 percent a year from 2006 through 2014, and by 16 percent a year from 2014 through 2017. Throughout this period, overdose rates were significantly higher for males (rising from 8.2 per 100,000 population in 1999 to 29.1 in 2017) than females (an increase from 3.9 in 1999 to 14.4 in 2017).

unethical—willing to overprescribe painkillers, or fill forged prescriptions, to make more money. Online pharmacies are particularly likely to violate the law: in 2016 the National Association of Boards of Pharmacy (NABP) reviewed 11,000 online drug outlets and concluded that 96 percent of them were not in compliance with the law and pharmacy industry standards.

Unethical physicians also play a role in the epidemic by overprescribing opioids. Doctors have strong financial reasons for supplying prescription painkillers out of their office. They can buy opioids wholesale, repackage them, and sell them to patients at a much higher price, with profits ranging from 60 to 300 percent. These illegal operations in which doctors, clinics or pharmacies prescribe or supply opioids without a legitimate medical reason are called "pill mills." To combat prescription opioid abuse, the DEA and some states have taken steps to eradicate pill mills.

TEXT-DEPENDENT QUESTIONS

1. What ancient Chinese doctor wrote the *Great Compendium of Herbs?*
2. How is trepanning performed?
3. Why were opioids created?

RESEARCH PROJECT

Look up the "Just Say No" anti-drug campaign from the 1980s online or in magazines. Find similar anti-drug policies and programs. Do you think these are an effective way to stop young people from using drugs? Write a brief essay about your opinion.

Hydrocodone is an opioid pain medication, derived from codeine, that is sold under the trade name Vicodin.

WORDS TO UNDERSTAND

endorphins—natural chemicals that the body releases that make people happy and feel less pain.

incompatible—two or more substances that cannot work together.

suppository—a solid medicine designed to be inserted into the rectum, where it melts.

CHAPTER 3

HOW OPIOID PAINKILLERS WORK

Over the past two decades, the most common way to treat chronic pain was to prescribe powerful drugs called opioid painkillers. The term *opioids* refers to an entire class of drugs that interacts with special receptors in the brain to produce painkilling effects. Some of these drugs are derived from a natural source, the opium poppy (*papaver somniferum*). These drugs, which include opium, morphine, and heroin, are part of the opioid class but are also known as opiates. Others were created in laboratories, rather than by processing opium, but they have the same painkilling effect on the brain. These opiates include painkillers like oxycodone, hydromorphone, and fentanyl.

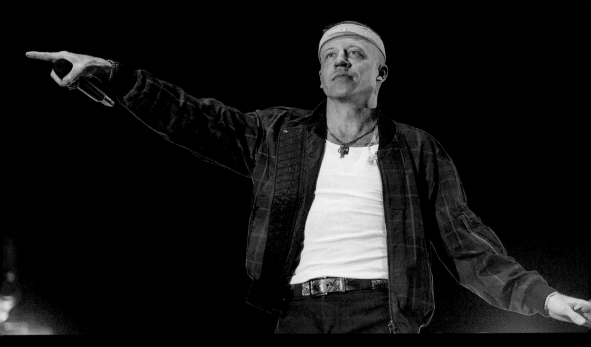

*In 2016, Rap star Macklemore discussed his addiction to OxyContin and other opioids on **Prescription for Change**, a documentary about the opioid crisis that aired on MTV.*

How Opioids Work

Opioid drugs are similar to chemicals that the brain and nervous system produce naturally. These chemicals, referred to as endogenous opioids, help the body control pain. They also release natural chemicals called **endorphins** which cause relaxation.

Within the brain, there are three types of opioid receptors. Scientists designate them as mu (μ), delta (δ), and kappa (κ) receptors. Each of these three receptors produces different effects in the body. When the receptors are activated by opioids, whether endogenous or synthetic, it triggers the release of certain chemicals into the body. Mu and delta receptors produce the pleasurable and pain-relieving effects of opioids. Kappa receptors play a role in the addictive properties of opioids.

Opioids act on three primary places in the brain and nervous system. The limbic system controls emotions. Here, opioids create sensations of pleasure, contentment, and ease. The brainstem is the source of automatic brain functions such as breathing. Here, opioids reduce pain, stop coughing, and slow down respiration. The spinal cord recognizes sensations from the body, then sends them to the brain. Opioids work in this area to decrease pain as well.

Eventually, the body naturally clears synthetic opioids from its systems. When that happens, the pain returns. More of the drugs must be taken to make pain recede again.

"Opioids trigger the release of endorphins, your brain's feel-good neurotransmitters," notes an informative article from the Mayo Clinic. "Endorphins muffle your perception of pain and boost feelings of pleasure, creating a temporary but powerful sense of well-being. When an opioid dose wears off,

To see a short video on how opioids work, scan here:

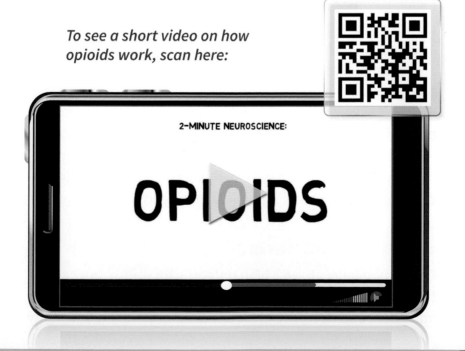

2-MINUTE NEUROSCIENCE:

OPIOIDS

you may find yourself wanting those good feelings back, as soon as possible. This is the first milestone on the path toward potential addiction."

Addiction and Tolerance

As opioids are used, the body and the brain gradually change. People who use opioid painkillers regularly develop a physical dependence on them. As a user's nervous system becomes used to regular doses of the drug, it stops naturally producing the endogenous opioids. This means the user must take larger amounts of the drug in order to achieve the same pain-relieving effects. This is called tolerance.

If the user tries to stop using an opioid, he or she will suffer from unpleasant physical effects, known as withdrawal. These generally include severe headaches, uncontrolled trembling, chills, pain and muscle spasms, insomnia, diarrhea, and vomiting. Some people experience nightmares, hallucinations, and depression. The symptoms of withdrawal can last for several weeks, and most people will do nearly anything to avoid them. This is a physical addiction.

"What makes opioid medications effective for treating pain can also make them dangerous," writes pharmacist Carry Krieger. "At lower doses, opioids may make you feel sleepy, but higher doses can slow your breathing and heart rate, which can lead to death. And the feelings of pleasure that result from taking an opioid can make you want to continue experiencing those feelings, which may lead to addiction."

Using Opioids Safely

Opioid painkillers have a high potential for abuse, but can be very effective in relieving chronic pain. Issues with abuse, addiction, and overdose generally stem from taking too many

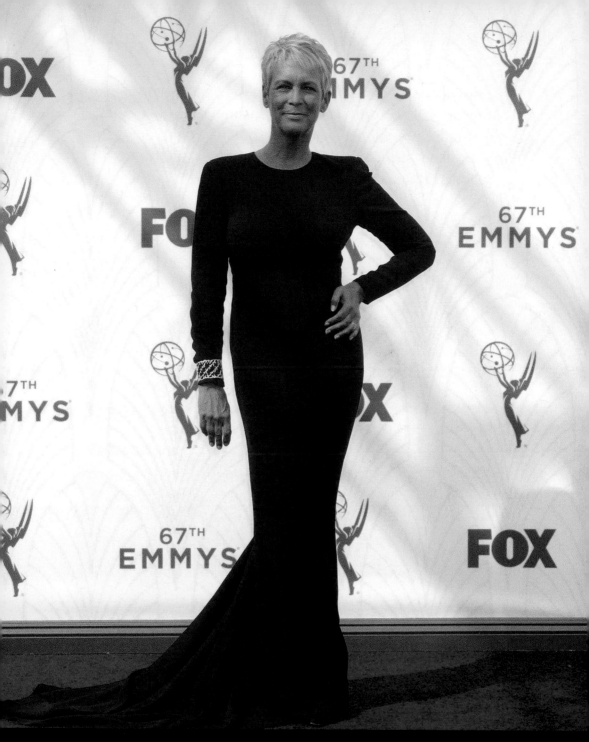

In 2018, movie star Jamie Lee Curtis admitted that she had become addicted to opioid painkillers after a surgical procedure. It took her ten years to quit using the powerful drugs.

prescription painkillers, taking them too often, or consuming them with illegal drugs, alcohol or **incompatible** medicines. Therefore, prescription painkillers should be taken only as prescribed, and for legitimate health reasons, such as to relieve chronic pain from surgery or an illness.

Upon getting a prescription filled, patients should check the label to ensure that it is the appropriate medication. If a measuring device is included in the prescription, instructions for using this tool should be followed precisely. Patients should never change the prescribed dosage without consulting their doctor first. They should also avoid taking medication that has been prescribed for someone else—this is especially important because the dose that is safe for the prescribed user may be deadly for someone else.

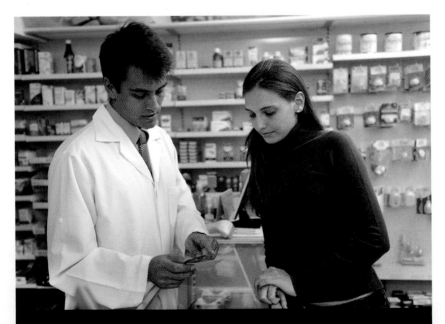

Federal laws require pharmacists to refuse to serve people they believe might be trying to purchase opioids with illegitimate prescriptions. The DEA provides guidance, in the form of specific warning signs, that pharmacists can use to determine whether or not to fill a prescription.

The FDA maintains a list of medicines that people should flush down the toilet immediately when they no longer need them, because they are too dangerous to leave around the house. Fentanyl, OxyContin, Demerol, and Vicodin are some of the common opioid painkillers on the "must flush" list. The full list is available at: https://www.fda.gov/downloads/drugs/resourcesforyou/consumers/buyingusingmedicinesafely/ensuringsafeuseofmedicine/safedisposalofmedicines/ucm337803.pdf

Law enforcement agencies sometimes hold "Drug Take-Back" days that allow the public to safely and anonymously discard medications, at no charge, no questions asked. These medications are often unused, unwanted, or expired. Such programs encourage individuals to dispose of their medications safely, while allowing law enforcement personnel to educate the public on opioid abuse. There is also an environmental benefit—medications are not being flushed down the toilet, which in rural areas can wind up affecting public water sources.

Before consuming prescription painkillers, patients should ask their doctor about the side effects and for any precautionary measures that they can take. For example, opioid use can cause drowsiness, so upon taking the medication, it is best not to drive or use any equipment that may cause injury. Patients taking other medicines or dietary supplements should tell their doctor before they start using prescription painkillers. They should also inform their physician if they are becoming dependent on or addicted to the drug.

Taking too many opiates can cause overmedication or overdose. Signs of overmedication include dizziness, confusion, slurred speech, stumbling while walking, extreme drowsiness, problems staying focused, and difficulty waking from sleep. Signs of overdose include inability to stay awake or speak; breathing problems such as slow, shallow breathing; lifelessness or limpness; blue fingernails or lips; clammy or pale skin; and stopped heartbeat. Opioid users and their family and friends should learn the signs of overmedication and overdose so they know how to respond in such situations.

Popular Opioid Painkillers

Morphine, which is derived from the opium poppy, is one of the most effective painkillers. It can be taken in oral doses, via **suppositories**, and intravenously. In addition to relieving pain, morphine also decreases hunger and reduces coughing. A related substance, codeine, has a milder effect and is used in some cough syrups. Hydrocodone is a drug that is derived from codeine. It is sold in pills, and sometimes combined with other non-opioid painkilling drugs, such as acetaminophen.

Hydromorphone is derived from morphine. It can be two to eight times more potent than morphine, though its effect does not last as long. The usual form of administration is by pills. In addition to reducing pain and suppressing coughing, the drug also produces feelings of euphoria, sedation, and relaxation. Hydromorphone is highly addictive both physically and psychologically.

During World War II, scientists created methadone in laboratories to combat a shortage of morphine. Today, the drug is most commonly used to help those addicted to heroin and other opioids control their withdrawal symptoms. Methadone binds with the opioid receptors but does not produce the same euphoric feelings as other opioids.

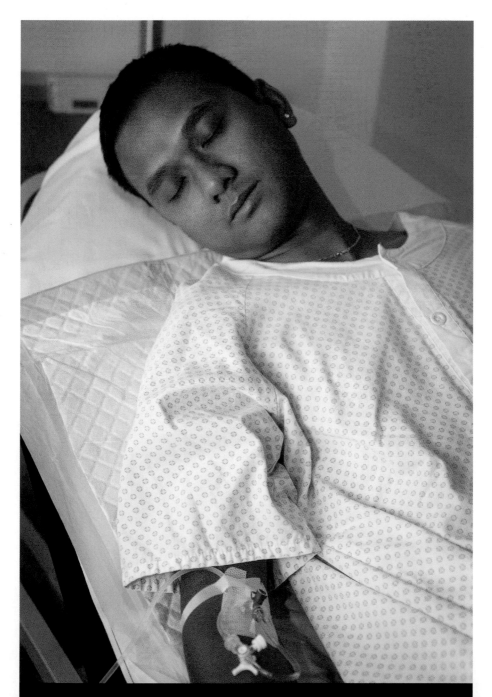

Morphine is often provided intravenously to control pain in patients who are recovering from surgery or a traumatic injury.

Oxycodone is among the most popular of the synthesized opioids. Under the brand name OxyContin, it has been widely abused. Oxycodone typically comes in pills, which are available in a variety of dosage strengths. Other pain-relieving products, such as aspirin or acetaminophen, have been effectively combined with oxycodone. The drug can also be taken via injection.

In 1949, Dr. Paul Janssen developed a synthetic opioid called fentanyl. Because it is eighty times more powerful than morphine, it became popular for pain relief. It is used in anesthetics, and also prescribed to help patients suffering from chronic cancer-related pain. Most patients are prescribed a fentanyl patch that transmits the drug through the skin, though the Actiq lollipop is also effective for long-term pain relief. Unfortunately, due to its potency fentanyl is often added to illegal street drugs like heroin, or to counterfeit opioid pills. Because of its potency it often results in deadly overdoses.

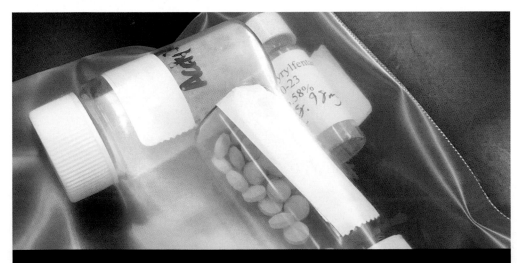

Illegal fentanyl pills, seized in a raid by the Drug Enforcement Agency (DEA). Of all the opioids available today, fentanyl is the strongest and deadliest. It does have legitimate medical uses as a painkiller, but it is regularly abused by drug addicts. Fentanyl's potency has contributed to the rise in opioid-related overdose deaths.

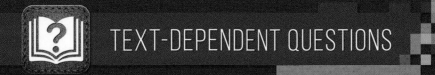

TEXT-DEPENDENT QUESTIONS

1. What are endorphins?
2. What are the three types of opioid receptors in the brain?
3. What morphine-related substance is used in some cough syrups?

RESEARCH PROJECT

By rereading the chapter and consulting reputable web pages and library books, compile a list of at least ten effects that opiates and opioids have on the body. Then, either print out a picture of a human body from the internet or draw one. Draw arrows to point out the areas affected.

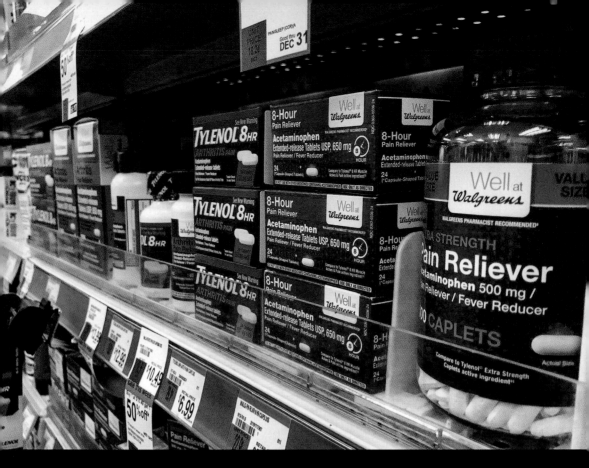

Over-the-counter pain medications are available in a variety of strengths and forms. Typically, both brand name and generic versions of over-the-counter drugs deliver a similar effect.

 WORDS TO UNDERSTAND

analgesic—a substance that relieves pain.

benzodiazepines—a class of drugs also called "tranquilizers," used to treat anxiety and some forms of pain. Include diazepam (Valium) and alprazolam (Xanax).

non-steroidal anti-inflammatory drug (NSAID)—a class of drugs used to treat mild to moderate pain. NSAID's include aspirin and ibuprofen.

CHAPTER 4

NON-OPIOID MEDICATIONS FOR PAIN

Although opioids are among the strongest pain relievers available today, there are many other accepted pain relieving drugs and substances. Some of these can be purchased "over the counter" at a local drugstore, or obtained through the internet. Others are only available with a doctor's prescription.

As concerns about the dangers of opioids grow, many physicians are seeking alternatives to these powerful painkillers. The good news is that studies indicate that, in the long term, non-opioid medications can be just as effective as opioid painkillers. "Treatment with opioids was not superior to treatment with nonopioid medications for improving pain-related function over 12 months," concluded a 2018 study published in the *Journal of the American Medical Association*. "Results do not support initiation of opioid therapy for moderate to severe chronic back pain or hip or knee osteoarthritis pain."

Over-the-Counter Drugs

Acetaminophen is an **analgesic** used to temporarily relieve minor aches and pains due to headache, muscular aches, backache, minor pain of arthritis, the common cold, toothache, and premenstrual and menstrual cramps. Acetaminophen is also used to temporarily reduce fever. Acetaminophen is sold under the brand name Tylenol, but

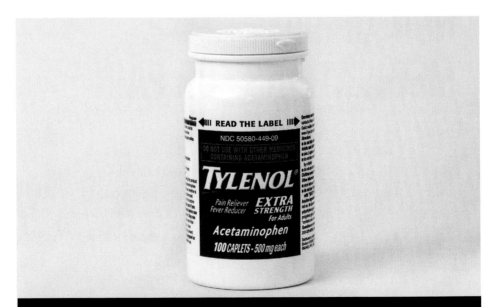

Requirements for drug packaging were tightened after 1982, when seven people in the Chicago area died from taking poisoned capsules that had been added to Tylenol bottles sitting on supermarket shelves. In response, the pharmaceutical industry developed sealed, tamper-resistant packaging, so that consumers could be sure that the drugs inside were safe.

many companies produce this pain reliever and it is often added to other medicines.

Over the counter versions of acetaminophen usually include less than 650 milligrams of the drug. A stronger prescription version called Ofirmev, delivered though an intravenous injection, was approved by the FDA in 2010. Ofirmev is prescribed for management of mild to moderate pain, and can be used along with certain opioids to treat moderate to severe pain.

Another prescription version combines acetaminophen with a mild opioid, codeine. Tylenol-Codeine contains 30 milligrams of codeine. Acetaminophen is not addictive by itself, but a person can develop an opioid addiction due to the codeine.

Another class of painkilling drugs are called **non-steroidal anti-inflammatory drugs**, or NSAIDs. These drugs lower inflammation, or swelling in the body, which puts pressure on

Scan here to learn more about NSAIDs:

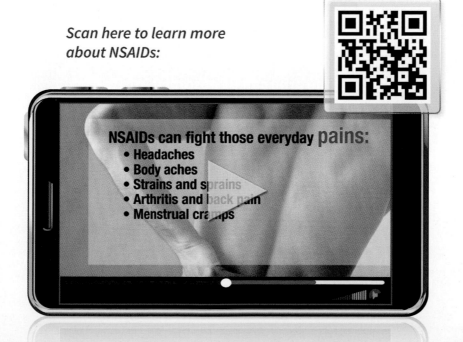

NSAIDs can fight those everyday pains:
- Headaches
- Body aches
- Strains and sprains
- Arthritis and back pain
- Menstrual cramps

SIDE EFFECTS OF NSAIDS

Although most people consider non-steroidal anti-inflammatory drugs like aspirin or ibuprofen to be extremely safe, these NSAIDs do sometimes cause serious side effects. In an article from *Everyday Health*, author Lynn Marks says these side effects are very rare, but they are something people should know about:

> NSAIDs can cause severe or life-threatening gastrointestinal (GI) bleeding and ulcers in some people. NSAIDs have also been linked to a higher risk of strokes, heart attacks, and heart-related deaths, especially when used for a long period of time. Additionally, the drugs can worsen high blood pressure, and may cause kidney damage in people over 60 years of age.

Other side effects include heartburn, gas, stomach pain, vomiting, and even headaches. Sometimes taking an NSAID with food or a glass of milk can avoid an upset stomach. The milk or food dilutes the drug and coats the stomach until the drug can be absorbed into the body.

Aspirin carries an additional risk for young people: Reye's syndrome. This is a rare condition that causes swelling in the liver and brain. This results in seizures and unconsciousness, and can cause permanent damage. Reye's syndrome often affects children or teenagers who are recovering from a viral infection such as the flu or chicken pox. The Mayo Clinic says that aspirin should never be given to children or teenagers who are recovering from these viral illnesses.

nerves, causing pain. NSAIDs prevent injured or damaged cells from releasing a chemical called prostaglandin, which helps carry pain messages through the nervous system. When the cells don't release this chemical, it means that the brain won't get the pain message as quickly or clearly. NSAIDs also reduce fevers, and can be combined with other drugs for increased effectiveness. Some are available over the counter, while other versions are available by prescription only.

The most common and oldest of the NSAIDs is aspirin. Despite thousands of years of use, aspirin is still tested by medical researchers to see why it works, how it works, and what unknown uses it might have. Today, aspirin is sold over the counter just about everywhere. Most aspirin today is synthetic, meaning it is made in a factory instead of being produced from willow tree bark.

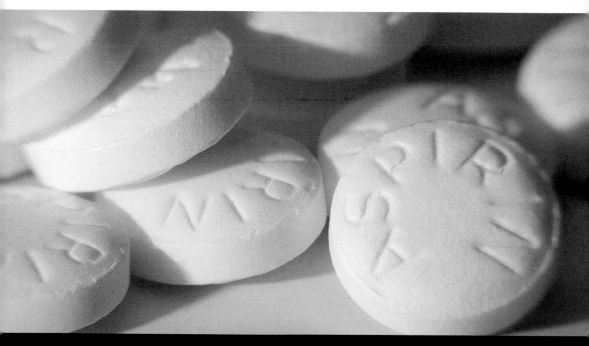

Aspirin is among the world's most popular painkillers, with roughly 100 billion tablets consumed each year.

Two other common over-the-counter NSAIDs are ibuprofen (sold as Motrin or Advil) and naproxen (sold as Aleve, Anaprox, Naprelan, or Naprosyn). Both of these drugs are also available as generic, store-branded versions.

OTC Supplements

People have been using herbal, vitamin, or mineral supplements to control pain for thousands of years. A supplement is something a person adds to his or her regular diet in hopes of getting positive health effects. Supplements often include ground-up plant leaves, roots, or bark—chewing on tree bark is how ancient people discovered willow tree bark reduced inflammation and reduced fevers.

Cannabidiol (CBD) has recently gathered a lot of attention for its supposed ability to ease pain, reduce anxiety, and provide other health benefits. The oil is derived from the cannabis (marijuana) plant, but does not make a person high; nor is it addictive. Its use has been approved by the FDA to treat certain types of epilepsy. Nora D. Volkow, the director of the National Institute on Drug Abuse, told Congress in 2015 that the substance might be an effective pain reliever. "In addition to epilepsy, the therapeutic potential of CBD is currently being explored for a number of indications including anxiety disorders, substance use disorders, schizophrenia, cancer, pain, inflammatory diseases and others," Volkow said.

Although research on the benefits of cannabidiol is incomplete, that has not stopped the substance from becoming a popular supplement. Because it is not regulated by the FDA, however, there is no oversight of the ways it is produced, or the amount of CBD that is in each supplement product. The consumer is left to read the label find out how much to take, when to take it, and how much of the active

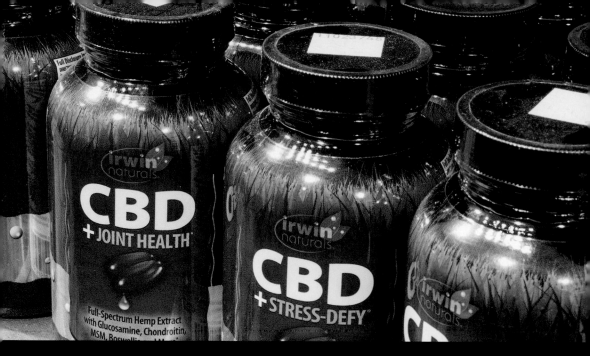

The popularity of CBD supplements have skyrocketed in recent years. Although CBD has been promoted as a cure for many ailments, its effectiveness has not yet been conclusively proven through scientific tests.

ingredient is in the product. Some products sold as hemp oil have very little CBD content.

Another supplement that claims to have pain-relieving benefits are the leaves of the kratom tree, which grows in southeast Asia. The supplement usually comes as a pill or a green powder; some people chew the leaves, or brew a tea with the powder to receive the effects. Kratom appears to interact with opioid receptors in the brain to decrease pain and produce a pleasant sensation, similar to other opioids. Another element in the leaves provides a stimulant effect.

Unlike other opioids, kratom is not illegal in the United States. However, because the plant's leaves can cause uncomfortable and sometimes dangerous side effects, government agencies have been closely monitoring its use over the past few years. In 2017, the Food and Drug Administration warned consumers about kratom. According

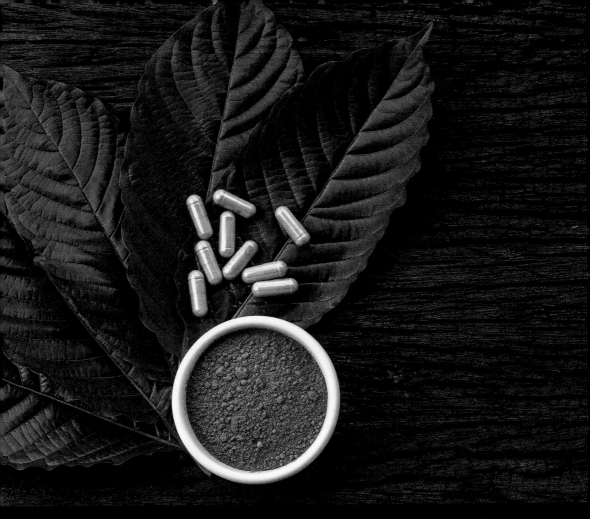

Leaves of the Mitragyna speciosa *tree, along with a bowl of the powdered product kratom, and capsules of the drug. This substance remains legal in the United States, although in recent years some federal drug officials have sought to ban its use.*

to the FDA, about 50 people have died from using kratom. In November 2018, the Department of Health and Human Services recommended that kratom be classified as a Schedule I substance, meaning that it has a high potential for abuse and no currently accepted medical use. This would make the supplement as illegal as heroin, marijuana, or other Schedule I drugs.

Muscle Relaxants

Benzodiazepines, sometimes called "tranquilizers" or "muscle relaxants," are a class of medications that work in the central nervous system. Benzodiazepines appear to work by dampening the activity of nerves in the brain and central nervous system. They are prescribed for a variety of medical conditions, including anxiety and seizures. They are effective at reducing acute pain, but don't work as well on chronic pain.

There are many types of benzodiazepines, which all have different strengths and durations. Some of the more popular include alprazolam (sold as Xanax), diazepam (Valium), and

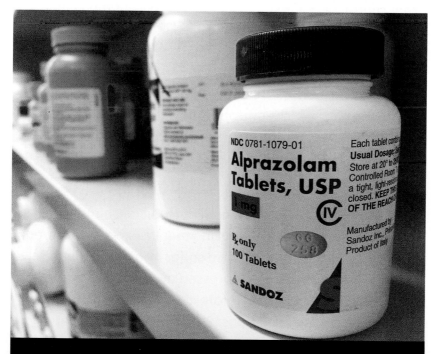

Benzodiazepines like alprazolam affect the body in a different way than opioids do. However, both benzodiazepines and opioids are commonly abused by recreational drug users, and both carry a high risk of fatal overdose.

lorazepam (Ativan). Some relaxers work directly on muscles, causing them to be less stiff and tense. Some work on the nerves, causing them to slow down or stop sending signals that tell muscles to tense up.

A side effect of this medication is sleepiness. That is why prescriptions advise people against driving, doing heavy work, and so forth while taking these drugs. When used in combination with opioids or alcohol, this effect is increased and can result in a fatal overdose due to respiratory depression.

"FDA is warning patients and their caregivers about the serious risks of taking opioids along with benzodiazepines or other central nervous system (CNS) depressant medicines, including alcohol," the agency warned in 2016. "Serious risks include unusual dizziness or lightheadedness, extreme sleepiness, slowed or difficult breathing, coma, and death. These risks result because both opioids and benzodiazepines impact the CNS, which controls most of the functions of the brain and body."

Antidepressants and Anticonvulsants

According to the Perelman School of Medicine, almost one-half of all primary care patients in America experience chronic pain. Many of these patients also suffer from major depressive disorder (MDD), which is a depressed mood that interferes with daily life. Suicide is therefore closely linked to people suffering from both conditions. Studies have found that people with chronic pain are twice as likely to commit suicide as those who are not suffering from chronic pain.

Perhaps because of this connection in the brain, some antidepressant medicines that help people deal with MDD are also used to treat certain kinds of pain. Researchers are not certain how these types of drugs work to reduce or eliminate pain caused by nerve damage. "The explicit way in which antidepressants are effective in pain management remains unknown, but multiple mechanisms are likely to be involved," write doctors Randy and Lori Sansone in a research paper published in the journal *Psychiatry*.

Anticonvulsants—medicines used to prevent seizures—are also sometimes used to treat pain caused by damage to the nervous system. Nerves that do not heal send constant pain signals to the brain. Somehow the anticonvulsants interrupt this signaling.

Gabapentin (sold as Gralise and Neurontin) and pregabalin (sold as Lyrica) are two modern medicines in this class that are often used to treat pain. They also have fewer side effects than older medicines in this category. The most common side effects are feeling sleepy and sometimes swelling in the legs.

Using anticonvulsants along with opioids is dangerous. Both types of medicine have the effect of depressing respiration, which can cause a person who takes too much to stop breathing.

Medical Marijuana

Since 1970, marijuana (*Cannabis sativa*) has been classified as an illegal Schedule I drug under the Controlled Substances Act. However, over the past few decades some medical researchers have worked to show that cannabis did in fact have legitimate medicinal uses. Numerous studies have shown that marijuana can be an effective pain reliever. A 2017 review of the medical literature by the National Academy of Sciences found that, "There is conclusive or substantial evidence that cannabis or cannabinoids are effective for the treatment of chronic pain in adults."

In 1996 California became the first state to legalize marijuana for limited purposes to manage chronic medical conditions. Today the use of medicinal marijuana is legal in thirty-three states, the District of Columbia, and Puerto Rico. All of these states allow doctors to prescribe medical marijuana to treat chronic pain. The presence of cannabidiol (CBD) in the marijuana is what relieves inflammation and pain, but the way it works is not well understood.

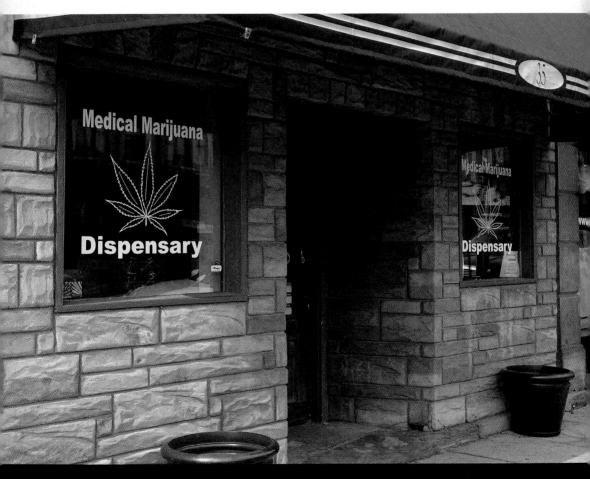

Medical marijuana dispensaries like this one in Michigan have become more common as states pass laws permitting the drug to be prescribed for treating certain conditions, including chronic pain.

TEXT-DEPENDENT QUESTIONS

1. What are two types of non-steroidal anti-inflammatory drugs?
2. How do kratom leaves work in the body?
3. What conditions are benzodiazepines prescribed to treat?

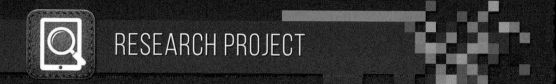

RESEARCH PROJECT

Using your school library, find out more about aspirin.
Write a one-page essay discussing the drug's history, uses,
common side effects, and dangers.

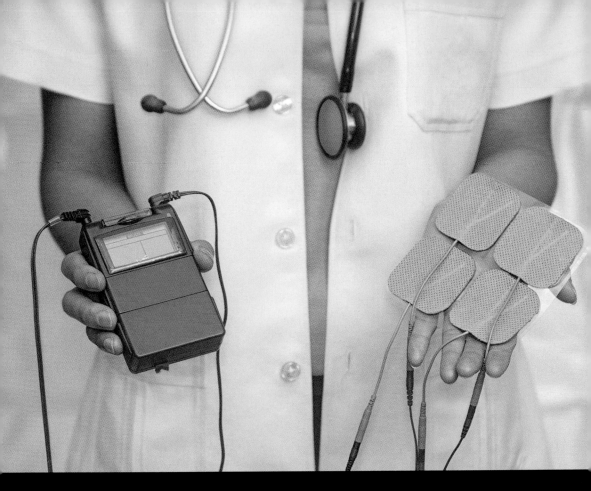

A doctor displays a transcutaneous electrical nerve stimulation (TENS) device. The patches are placed on the skin in the area where pain is felt, and a mild electrical pulse from the device stimulates the nerve endings and relieves pain.

WORDS TO UNDERSTAND

migraine—a severe headache, which is very painful and makes the person extremely sensitive to noise and light.

transcranial—something that passes through the skull into the brain.

transcutaneous—through the skin.

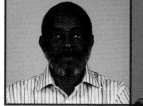

CHAPTER 5

ALTERNATIVE THERAPIES

While drugs are the most common way to treat pain, there are many other ways to deal with pain. As the opioid crisis continues to destroy lives, alternative therapies for pain relief continue to grow. Some popular methods involve ancient practices; others are modern concepts. Some of these alternative therapies are widely accepted and others are not. Most of these ideas continue to be studied by medical science.

As scientific understanding of pain evolves, doctors are more willing to accept these alternative pain relief methods. "That phrase 'alternative pain treatments' doesn't mean much to me," comments Dr. Seddon R. Savage, a former president of the American Pain Society. "I think the line between them and mainstream treatment is pretty blurry now."

Here are some modern pain relief alternatives to opioids.

Acupuncture

Acupuncture is an ancient Chinese method of relieving pain and treating disease by inserting needles into specific areas of the body. Acupuncturists believe that every person has a life force that flows through their body, called *qi*. Pain and disease are caused when the *qi* is blocked or out of balance. Acupuncture is a method of placing very thin needles at precise points on the body to redirect the *qi* and allow healing.

"Each acupuncture needle produces a tiny injury at the insertion site, and although it's slight enough to cause little to no discomfort, it's enough of a signal to let the body know it needs to respond," explains Paul Kempisty, a licensed acupuncturist. "This response involves stimulation of the

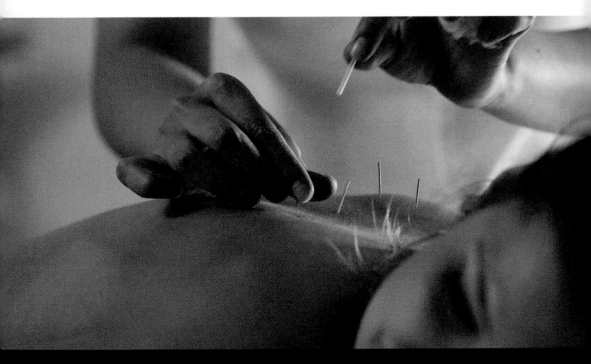

Acupuncture is an ancient Chinese healing practice, but modern scientific studies have found that it can help ease some types of chronic pain and relieve or prevent headaches.

ACUPUNCTURE NEEDLES

Some people who aren't familiar with acupuncture may be scared by the idea of needles being pushed into their skin. Others are not bothered. For those who can overcome a fear of needles, acupuncture may provide relief from pain.

Most acupuncture needles are made in China, Japan, and Korea. Their quality and standards can vary, which some researchers believe is a problem. In the United States, the Food and Drug Administration (FDA) sets certain requirements for acupuncture needles, just as it does for the medical needles used to inject medicines or vaccinations. The FDA says the acupuncture needles should only be used once, should be sterilized after each use, and should be made from bio-compatible materials that have been shown not to affect people in a negative way. Stainless steel is the most common material for acupuncture needles, but occasionally gold or silver needles are used. Acupuncture needles can be long or short. The part that pierces the skin is always very thin, from 0.27 to 0.46 millimeters—about ten times as thick as a human hair.

immune system, promoting circulation to the area, wound healing, and pain modulation."

Practiced throughout Asia and Europe, acupuncture has gained acceptance with many people in the United States and Canada. Some members of the medical profession find that acupuncture is useful as a helpful, additional treatment to other Western medicines; others find it to be an acceptable alternative in its own right. Most US states and Canadian provinces regulate and grant licenses to establishments that offer acupuncture.

Chiropractic

Chiropractic care is based on the idea that the musculoskeletal system, particularly the spine, plays an important role in the body's health. When the vertebrae in the spine are out of line, this causes problems, including pain. The goal of chiropractic care is put the spinal vertebrae back into proper alignment.

Chiropractors may include other therapies in treatment that include learning how to avoid problems that cause back pain, notes a recent report from Harvard Medical School. "While the mainstay of chiropractic is spinal manipulation, chiropractic care may also include other treatments, including manual or manipulative therapies, postural and exercise education, and ergonomic training (how to walk, sit, and stand to limit back strain)," the report explains. "Chiropractors today often work in conjunction with primary care doctors, pain experts, and surgeons to treat patients with pain."

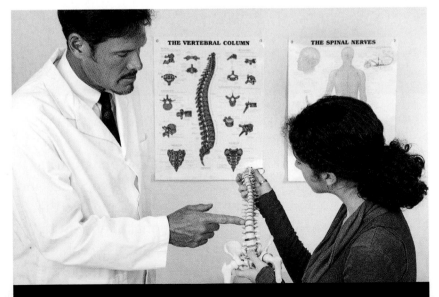

A chiropractor uses a model of the spine while discussing treatment with a patient.

Electricity and Magnetism

The use of electrical impulses to relieve pain is a practice that can be traced to ancient times. In ancient Egypt, healers used to catch electric eels in the Nile River and lay them over the wounds of patients. In the eighteenth century, the scientist Benjamin Franklin, who experimented with electricity using primitive batteries called Leyden jars, came to believe that mild electrical shocks could relieve pain.

Today, a method called **transcutaneous** electrical nerve stimulation (TENS) is a popular treatment for lower back pain and arthritis aches. A TENS unit uses small disks to transmit an electrical charge through the skin to muscles and nerves underneath. The electrical charge is low and the sensation is not supposed to be painful. The disk is held in place with a mild adhesive. TENS units are common in physical therapy clinics. Some people suffering from chronic pain have their own TENS units which they use as needed.

Scan here to see how a TENS unit works:

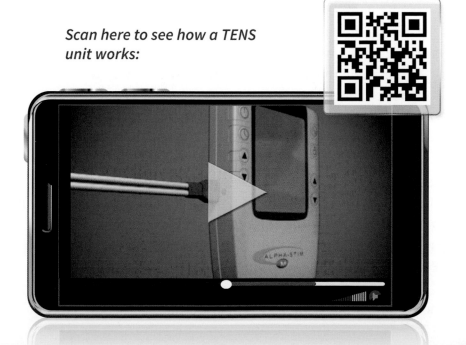

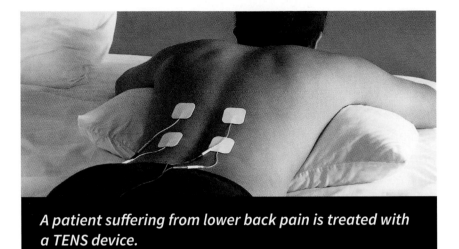

A patient suffering from lower back pain is treated with a TENS device.

Magnetism is a form of electricity, but one that does not deliver an electrical shock. Using magnets to control pain goes back thousands of years and was used around the world. The ancient Greeks, Egyptians, and Chinese used magnets for healing, as did the native people of Mesoamerica. In the sixteenth century the Swiss alchemist Paracelsus reasoned that since magnets had the power to attract iron, perhaps they could also attract diseases and remove them from the body.

Permanent magnets are materials that have a natural magnetic charge. Lodestones are a common type of naturally occurring magnet. Some people believe wearing jewelry made from natural magnets, such as lodestones, or from conductive minerals like copper, can help relieve pain. However, modern researchers have not been able to conclusively prove whether these types of magnets are effective for treating pain. "Scientific studies on human subjects have failed to show the efficacy of using magnets to treat pain or joint and muscle stiffness," writes Elizabeth Palermo, associate editor at *Live Science*.

However, there are some studies that indicate magnets do hold some promise for pain relief. "Some studies have shown that magnetic fields may cause changes in nerve cell function, which in turn blocks pain signals," writes Sara Calabro. "Other theories are that magnets may offer pain relief by causing an increase in blood flow and oxygen to tissues, or that magnetic pain therapy works by balancing the death and growth of cells. Increased body temperature also may play a role in how magnets bring about pain relief."

Unlike permanent magnets, electromagnets require an electrical charge to be active. The National Institutes of Health has found that electromagnets are effective at treating some kinds of pain, such as arthritis. In 2013 the FDA approved a device that uses strong electromagnets to treat **migraines** by stimulating nerve cells in the brain, a process called **transcranial** magnetic stimulation (TMS). In recent years, the National Institutes of Health has reported that TMS may help other pain conditions as well.

Exercise

When movement causes pain, as in the case of arthritis, it seems counterintuitive that moving even more could help to ease that pain. But arthritis pain responds well to certain types of exercise, as long as it's done properly. "[T]he right set of exercises can be a long-lasting way to tame ankle, knee, hip, or shoulder pain," noted a post on the Harvard Medical School's blog HealthBeat. "Practiced regularly, joint pain relief workouts might permit you to postpone—or even avoid—surgery on a problem joint that has been worsening for years by strengthening key supportive muscles and restoring flexibility."

Low-impact exercises include walking, aerobics, Pilates, tai chi, and yoga. Walking is regularly listed as one of the best exercises, because it can be done anywhere and at any time, without requiring any special training or equipment. Water aerobics are the same as aerobics on land, done in chest-deep water.

Yoga is an ancient form of exercise, originating in South Asia, that is based around performing different poses or postures. It can help practitioners build strength and flexibility. A meditative focus on breathing can help people to improve their mental state as well. There are many different styles of yoga. Yoga has become so accepted that some insurance companies will now pay for classes when they are prescribed by a doctor.

Tai chi was originally created by Buddhist monks in China as a form of martial arts. Today, like yoga, it is practiced as a health-promoting, low-impact activity. Research has suggested that tai chi can help reduce stress levels, improve

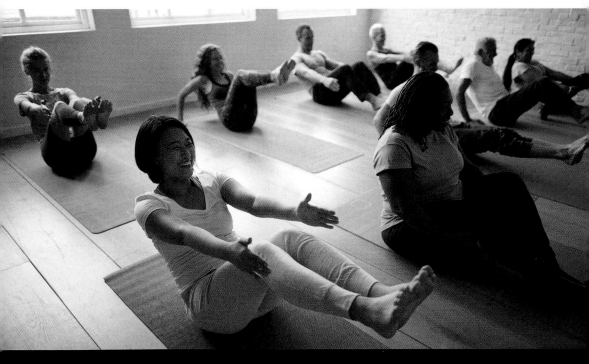

Low-impact fitness programs like yoga or tai chi can help to relieve pain.

balance, increase muscle strength in your legs, and improve general mobility and flexibility.

Unlike yoga and tai chi, Pilates was developed in the early twentieth century by a German physical trainer named Joseph Pilates. He developed a method of physical fitness that on strengthening the body through exercises, often utilizing weights or resistance bands. The health benefits of Pilates can include improved posture and better balance and mobility, and there is some evidence that suggests Pilates can beneficial for those who suffer from back pain.

Training the Mind

Because pain is connected to the nervous system and the brain, pain can literally be said to be a matter of mind. Some non-drug therapies try to teach people how to use their mind to control pain. Meditation, psychotherapy, and hypnosis are the three most common methods.

Through meditation, a person is able to achieve a mentally clear, emotionally calm state. One technique useful for meditation is called mindfulness—focusing the mind on a particular object, thought, or activity to train attention and awareness. Meditation can actually create physical changes in the brain. A 2014 study published in the *Journal of the American Medical Association* found that meditation can lead to pain relief, and also help people fight opioid addiction.

Psychotherapy is the process of talking out problems with a trained therapist, who guides the discussion so the person seeking help gets the most from each session. Psychotherapy does not treat the source of physical pain. Instead, can help people find ways to deal with pain. This kind of pain relief is especially helpful for mental and emotional pain, both of which can drive people to opioid abuse to find relief.

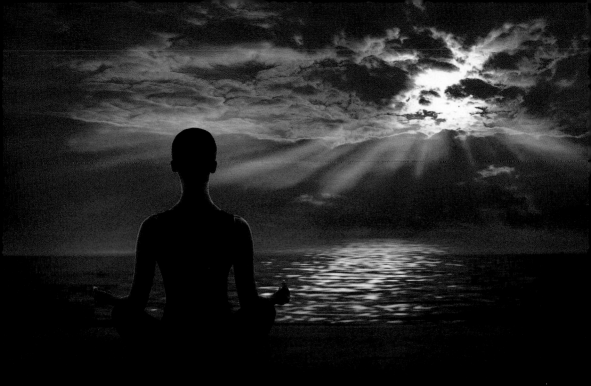

Some people have succeeded at keeping pain at bay through meditation, or by natural methods such as changing their diet, losing weight, and exercising.

Hypnosis is another form of training the mind to control addictive behaviors and some kinds of pain. In hypnosis, the patient is put into a relaxed trace state, where they are open to suggestions and experience heightened imagination. Not everyone can be hypnotized; those who can, however, have shown some promise of pain relief. A small study in Israel showed hypnosis has some promise in helping people overcome opioid addiction. The study also said much more research is needed, however.

Alternative therapies sometimes work, sometimes don't and sometimes cause problems greater than the pain they are supposed to treat. Alternate therapies should be used with caution.

TEXT-DEPENDENT QUESTIONS

1. What is acupuncture?
2. How does chiropractic care ease pain?
3. What are some differences between yoga, tai chi and pilates?

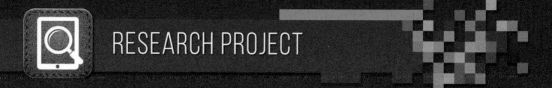

RESEARCH PROJECT

Using the internet or your school library, find out more about how electrical impulses can be used to treat pain. Is electrical therapy effective for all kinds of pain? If not, what kinds of pain does it help control most effectively? Write a one-page paper and present it to your class.

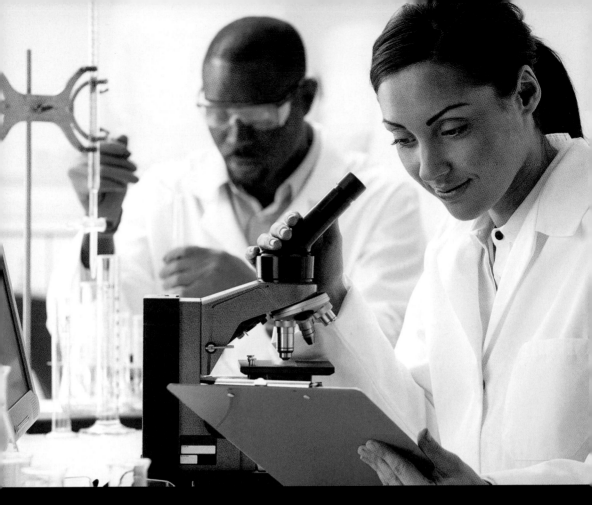

Creating a new painkilling drug requires years of research and testing.

 WORDS TO UNDERSTAND

ablation—using electricity to burn away cells in a body that are causing health problems.

platelet—a type of cell found in blood and bone marrow that helps with blood clotting and healing.

protein—a string of amino acids that make up parts of every living thing on earth.

CHAPTER 6

EXPERIMENTAL TREATMENTS

Medical science is always looking for new and better ways to treat pain. Scientists are constantly creating new synthetic compounds, as well as examining previously unused plants and animals, to see if they can have beneficial health effects. Some of these substances hold the promise of effective pain relief without the high risk of addiction that comes with opioids.

Preventing addiction is a driving reason behind much of the research. "With more than 100 Americans dying from opioid overdoses every day, there is an urgent need for drugs that offer strong pain-relieving properties without leading to addiction," says an article on the website Science Daily.

Most of these potential drugs will never make it into pharmacies, or help people in pain. Some may turn out to have side effects that are worse than opioids. Some may be

Getting any new drug to the marketplace in the United States means complying with research and testing procedures established by the Food and Drug Administration. When a pharmaceutical company develops a new drug, there is no guarantee it will ever be approved for human use. It usually takes at least ten to twelve years for a drug to be approved for widespread human use via prescription. According to the Bloomberg School of Public Health, the average total cost of developing a new drug is estimated at $2 billion to $3 billion.

When a pharmaceutical company wants to bring a useful new drug to market, it applies to the FDA to begin testing. The first round of tests are conducted on research mice or other animals. If these initial tests indicate that the drug will probably be safe for humans, experimental human trials are scheduled. Phase I tests utilize a very small number of people (twenty to eighty). The goal is to determine how the drug reacts in the body, and to identify side effects. Next are Phase II tests, which involve a few hundred people and are meant to determine how well the drug works on a particular condition or disease.

At the end of Phase II, the FDA and pharmaceutical company plan how large-scale Phase III studies, involving thousands of people, will be conducted. These studies gather more information about the safety and effectiveness of the drug, study different populations and different dosages, and use the drug in combination with other drugs.

When the testing is complete, a new drug application is filed with the FDA. The application includes all data from the testing, as well as information about how the drug will be manufactured and labeled. The FDA assigns a team of doctors, statisticians, chemists, pharmacologists, and other scientists to review the test data and proposed label. It also inspects the factory where the drug will be made.

Even after the FDA approves a drug for sale to the public, the oversight continues. The FDA's monitoring process may uncover problems that were not observed in the pre-approval trials. If the problems are serious enough, the FDA can decide that the drug cannot be sold anymore.

too dangerous for other reasons. These new drugs are also years away from being available to people in pain. It often takes more than a decade for a proposed new drug to move from the laboratory where it was created into trials that test its effects on real people. Sometimes several rounds of human tests are required before a pharmaceutical company receives approval from the Food and Drug Administration to begin marketing and selling a new product.

In 2018, the FDA announced plans to reduce the time and experimental trials needed to get alternative pain medicines to market. This decision was promoted by the opioid epidemic, according to an article in the *Washington Post*. "As part of the effort, the agency plans to withdraw its existing 2014 guidance to the drug industry on pain medicines," writes *Post* reporter Laurie McGinley. "That document is overly broad, [FDA Commissioner Scott] Gottlieb said, and is sometimes a barrier to new products and innovations. The current guidelines call for a large number of studies to get FDA approval for general use for chronic pain."

Making Safer Opioids

Some researchers are trying to make synthetic opioids less addictive. The idea is to make an effective opioid that does not lead to addiction, but still stops pain. In 2017 the American College of Neuropsychopharmacology reported that Dr. Laura Bohn and other scientists at the Scripps Research Institute "may have found a way to make opioids safer by separating the drugs' pain-relieving effects from their most dangerous side effect, respiratory suppression, which, in very severe cases, causes patients to stop breathing and to die." The experimental medicine works by only stimulating the opioid receptors to stimulate pain relief, but providing less stimulation of the pathway that leads to respiratory suppression.

Another group of researchers is working on painkillers that naturally mimic the body's own pain-relieving chemicals and interact with opioid receptors, but don't result in addiction. The group, from the University of Michigan, revealed their progress in a 2018 article in the journal *Experimental Biology*. "Our hope is that with our novel opioids, patients would need less of the drug over time, which might put them less at risk for the negative side effects of opioid usage, including addiction, respiratory depression and constipation," said research team member Nicholas Griggs. The new drugs have been tested in mice, but not yet in human trials.

The US government is also putting money into non-addictive opioid research. In September of 2018, Phoenix Pharma Labs received a $2.7 million grant from the US Department of Defense to further research a new drug called PPL-103. This experimental drug activates all three opioid receptors in the brain (mu, kappa and delta), but only stimulates them partially. The theory is that this is enough for the receptors to release pain-relieving chemicals, but not enough to produce the stronger side effects of other opioids. The Department of Defense is interested in this research because veterans are at higher risk of addiction and substance abuse than the general population.

New Technologies and Therapies

In addition to improved drugs, a variety of new technologies offer the prospect of relief for people living with chronic pain. One of these technologies is radiofrequency **ablation** (RFA). An electrical current produced by a radio wave is used to heat up a small area of nerve tissue. This results in decreased pain

VARICOSE VEINS TREATMENT WITH RADIOFREQUENCY ABLATION or OBLITERATION

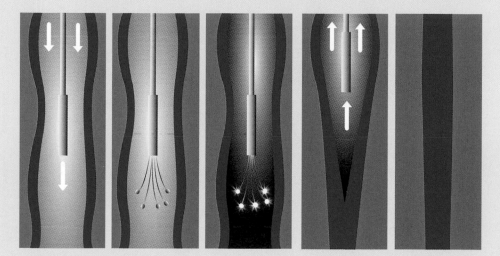

Catheter inserted into the vein   Electrodes are placed in the vein   A radiofrequency wave is sent   Catheter withdrawn, closing vein   Closed vein following treatment

This diagram shows how radiofrequency ablation is used to treat varicose veins. The procedure uses heat to kill nerve tissue, providing relief from pain. It has been shown effective for treating spinal arthritis and nerve damage, as well as to destroy tumors.

signals from that area. RFA treatments are effective about 70 percent of the time, and the analgesic effect can last for six months or longer.

Another approach involves the electrical stimulation of the spinal cord. A small device is implanted in the patient's back, and attached to the spinal cord. By pressing a button, the patient causes the device to deliver low-power electrical pulses. These pulses interfere with the pain messages sent by nerves, preventing them from reaching the brain. Although it is growing more common, spinal cord stimulation is generally only used when more conventional treatments or surgery have failed to work.

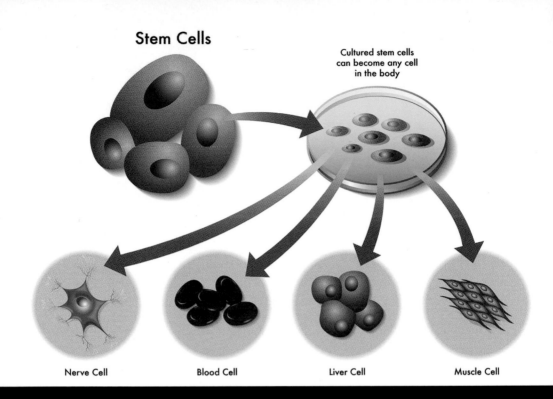

Stem Cells

Cultured stem cells
can become any cell
in the body

Nerve Cell   Blood Cell   Liver Cell   Muscle Cell

Stem cells could play an important role in pain relief because of their ability to become any type of cell in the human body.

One promising research area involves harvesting stem cells from a patient's bone marrow and injecting them into an area, such as the lower back, that has become painful because tissue has deteriorated. Stem cells are unusual because of their versatility—they can become brain, organ, blood, or bone cells as needed. The theory behind this treatment is that the stem cells can build new, healthy tissue in the damaged areas, and eliminate the pain for good. Since 2015, experimental treatments have yielded good results, but much more research is needed. "Though the data from existing studies look promising for the use of stem cells as a novel therapeutic strategy for [pain], additional clinical studies will be needed to validate the benefit of the technology for clinical use," noted a 2017 study in the journal *Pain Physician*.

Some medical clinics offer different treatments that utilize the injection of bodily fluids or tissue extracts into painful areas. Sometimes these treatments include stem cells, and sometimes not. Some clinics use untested methods of drawing stem cells from the patient's body fat, rather than from bone marrow. The clinics advertise that these treatments provide a quick and permanent cure for pain caused by arthritis, nerve damage, or degenerative conditions. However, the FDA has not approved these treatments, and warns that there is no evidence that they have any beneficial long-term effects.

One of the best-known of these experimental technologies is called **platelet**-rich plasma therapy. It involves drawing blood from a patient, spinning it in a centrifuge to produce a high concentration of platelet cells, and then injecting this solution into a damaged joint, such as a knee. Some high-profile athletes, including Kobe Bryant, Peyton Manning, and Tiger Woods have used this therapy in hopes of prolonging their careers.

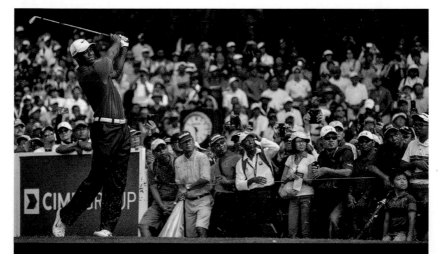

Golf star Tiger Woods underwent platelet-rich plasma therapy treatments to help reduce the pain of a knee injury that threatened to derail his career.

From Poison to Pain Relief

For some people, the idea of being bitten by a poisonous snake or reptile is simply terrifying. However, researchers have found that some of the substances in venom may hold the key to pain relief. That sounds odd, given that bites from venomous creatures cause pain. However, scientists have been able to take venom and remove the deadly elements that are meant to kill prey animals quickly.

Medicines derived from snake venoms are also used for other medical purposes. Captopril, for example, is based on the venom of pit vipers (like rattlesnakes) and used to treat high blood pressure and other heart problems. The Food and Drug Administration has approved at least five other drugs made from venoms; many more are currently being tested.

To see a snake being "milked" of venom, scan here:

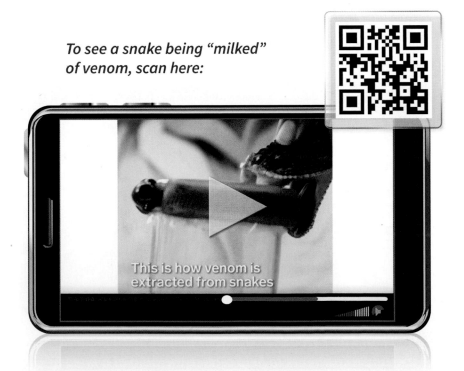

This is how venom is extracted from snakes

The black mamba (Dendroaspis polylepis) derives its name from the dark coloration inside its mouth; the snake's skin color usually varies from dull yellowish-green to a gun-metal grey. These deadly snakes are native to Africa.

The black mamba is one of the world's deadliest snakes; a bite can kill a person in just a few hours. Yet in 2012, researchers found that certain **proteins** isolated from black mamba venom, called mambalgins, are actually potent painkillers. "When it was tested in mice, the analgesia was as strong as morphine, but you don't have most of the side-effects," Dr. Eric Lingueglia of the Institute of Molecular and Cellular Pharmacology in France told the BBC. "It is the very first stage, of course, and it is difficult to tell if it will be a painkiller in humans or not. A lot more work still needs to be done in animals."

Another area of research is the venomous cone snail. There are roughly 600 cone snail species found in undersea habitats around the world, but the *Conus regius*, found in the Caribbean, is currently being studied by scientists at the

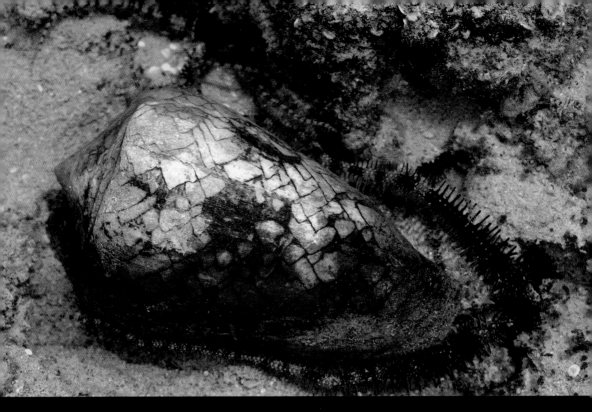

The venom of the crown cone snail (Conus regius), a small marine animal found in the Caribbean Sea, is capable of paralyzing and killing prey. It may also provide long-term pain relief in humans.

University of Utah. This snail's venom appears to stop pain for an extended period, and may even boost the body's ability to repair damaged nerves.

"We found that the compound was still working 72 hours after the injection, still preventing pain," said J. Michael McIntosh, a professor of psychiatry at the University of Utah Health Sciences. "What is particularly exciting about these results is the aspect of prevention. Once chronic pain has developed, it is difficult to treat. This compound offers a potential new pathway to prevent chronic pain from developing in the first place and also offers a new therapy to patients with established pain who have run out of options."

TEXT-DEPENDENT QUESTIONS

1. What are some barriers to getting new pain medications to market?
2. What are some side effects of non-opioid pain relievers?
3. What is platelet-rich plasma therapy?

RESEARCH PROJECT

Write a one-page essay about migraines. Find someone who experiences migraines and ask them about their pain. Some questions to ask are: What causes a migraine? How does the person treat a migraine? What part of the head is most affected? Talk to a pharmacist and ask what prescription drugs can treat migraines. List your information sources at the end of the essay.

CHAPTER NOTES

CHAPTER 1

p. 7:   "the unpleasant sensory and emotional experience …" International Association for the Study of Pain, "IASP Terminology" (December 14, 2017). https://www.iasp-pain.org/Education/Content.aspx?ItemNumber=1698

p. 7:   "Pain is an unpleasant …" Adam Felman, "What is pain and how do you treat it?" *Medical News Today* (July 27, 2017). https://www.medicalnewstoday.com/articles/145750.php

p. 15:   "Research shows that women …" Craig Freudenrich, "How Pain Works," How Stuff Works (November 9, 2007). https://science.howstuffworks.com/life/inside-the-mind/human-brain/pain3.htm

p. 15:   "Central post-stroke pain …" National Stroke Association, "Pain" (accessed February 25, 2019). https://www.stroke.org/we-can-help/survivors/stroke-recovery/post-stroke-conditions/physical/pain/

p. 18:   "There's no way I could live …" Steven Pete, quoted in Erika Hayasaki, "End Pain Forever: How a Single Gene Could Become a Volume Knob for Pain," *Wired* (April 18, 2017). https://www.wired.com/2017/04/the-cure-for-pain/

CHAPTER 2

p. 23:   "People have used alcohol …" National Institute on Alcohol Abuse and Alcoholism, "Using Alcohol to Relieve Your Pain: What Are the Risks?" (July 2013). https://pubs.niaaa.nih.gov/publications/PainFactsheet/Pain_alcohol.pdf

CHAPTER 3

p. 37:   "Opioids trigger the release …" Mayo Clinic staff, "How Opioid Addiction Occurs," The Mayo Clinic (February 26, 2018). https://www.mayoclinic.org/diseases-conditions/prescription-drug-abuse/in-depth/how-opioid-addiction-occurs/art-20360372

p. 38:   "What makes opioid medications effective …" Carrie Krieger, "What are Opioids and Why Are they Dangerous?" The Mayo Clinic (accessed February 25, 2019). https://www.mayoclinic.org/diseases-conditions/prescription-drug-abuse/expert-answers/what-are-opioids/faq-20381270

CHAPTER 4

p. 47:   "Treatment with opioids was not …" Erin E. Krebs et al., "Effect of Opioid vs Nonopioid Medications on Pain-Related Function in Patients With Chronic Back Pain or Hip or Knee Osteoarthritis Pain," *Journal of the American Medical Association* 319, no. 9 (March 6, 2018). https://jamanetwork.com/journals/jama/fullarticle/2673971

p. 50:   "NSAIDs can cause severe …" Lynn Marks, "What are NSAIDs?" Everyday Health (October 16, 2015). https://www.everydayhealth.com/nsaid/guide/

p. 52:   "In addition to epilepsy …" Nora D. Volkow, "The Biology and Potential Therapeutic Effects of Cannabidiol," testimony before the Senate Caucus on International Narcotics Control (June 24, 2015). https://www.drugabuse.gov/about-nida/legislative-activities/testimony-to-congress/2015/biology-potential-therapeutic-effects-cannabidiol

p. 56:   "FDA is warning patients …" FDA Drug Safety Communication (August 31, 2016). https://www.fda.gov/Drugs/DrugSafety/ucm518473.htm

p. 57:   "The explicit way in which …" Randy A. Sansone and Lori A. Sansone, "Pain, Pain, Go Away," *Psychiatry* 5, no. 12 (December 2008). https://www.ncbi.nlm.nih.gov/pmc/articles/PMC2729622/pdf/PE_5_12_16.pdf

p. 57:   "There is conclusive or substantial …" The National Academies of Sciences, *The Health Effects of Cannabis and Cannabinoids* (Washington, DC: National Academies Press, 2017), p. 13.

CHAPTER 5

p. 61:   "That phrase 'alternative pain treatments' …" Seddon R. Savage, quoted in David A. Bohn, *The Unconventional Guide to Reversing Pain* (New York: Lulu, 2017), p. 10.

p. 62:   "Each acupuncture needle …" Paul Kempisty, quoted in Danielle Sinay, "Is Acupuncture the Miracle Remedy for Everything?" *Health Line* (November 30, 2017). https://www.healthline.com/health/acupuncture-how-does-it-work-scientifically#how-does-it-work

CHAPTER NOTES

p. 64:   "While the mainstay of chiropractic …" Harvard Health Publishing, "Chiropractic Care for Pain Relief," Harvard Medical School (June 6, 2018). https://www.health.harvard.edu/pain/chiropractic-care-for-pain-relief

p. 66:   "Scientific studies on human subjects …" Elizabeth Palermo, "Does Magnetic Therapy Work?" Live Science (February 11, 2015). https://www.livescience.com/40174-magnetic-therapy.html

p. 66:   "Some studies have shown …" Sara Calabro, "Do Magnets Offer Pain Relief?" *Everyday Health* (July 27, 2010). https://www.everydayhealth.com/alternative-health/treatment-regimens/use-of-magnets-for-pain.aspx

p. 67:   "[T]he right set of exercises …" Harvard Health Publishing, "The Joint Pain Relief Workout: Healing Exercises for your Shoulders, Hips, Knees, and Ankles," Harvard Medical School (September 23, 2013). https://blog.content.health.harvard.edu/blog/special-reports/the-joint-pain-relief-workout-healing-exercises-for-your-shoulders-hips-knees-and-ankles/

CHAPTER 6

p. 73:   "With more than 100 Americans …" Experimental Biology, "Promise for Safer Opioid Pain Reliever: New Compound Offers Pain-Relief of Opioids without Tolerance or Addictive properties," *Science Daily* (April 23, 2018). www.sciencedaily.com/releases/2018/04/180423155043.htm

p. 75:   "As part of the effort …" Laurie McGinley, "FDA Pushes for Development of Non-opioid Pain Medications," *Washington Post* (August 29, 2018). https://www.washingtonpost.com/news/to-your-health/wp/2018/08/29/fda-pushes-for-development-of-non-opioid-pain-medications/

p. 75:   "may have found a way …" American College of Neuropsychopharmacology, "Safer Opioid Drugs Could Treat Pain and Save Lives," *Science Daily* (December 5, 2017). www.sciencedaily.com/releases/2017/12/171205091537.htm

p. 76:   "Our hope is that …" Nicholas Griggs, quoted in "Promise for Safer Opioid Pain Reliever." Science Daily (accessed March 12, 2019). www.sciencedaily.com/releases/2018/04/180423155043.htm.

p. 78:   "Though the data from existing studies …" Paul J. Christo, et al. "Stem Cell Therapy for Chronic Pain Management: Review of Uses, Advances, and Adverse Effects," *Pain Physician* 20, no 4 (May/June 2017), p. 293. https://www.painphysicianjournal.com/current/pdf?article=NDQwNg%3D%3D&journal=105

p. 81:   "When it was tested in mice …" Dr. Eric Lingueglia, quoted in James Gallagher, "Black Mamba Venom is 'Better Painkiller" than Morphine," BBC News (October 3, 2012). https://www.bbc.com/news/health-19812064

p. 82:   "We found that the compound …" J. Michael McIntosh, quoted in Stacy Kish, "An Alternative to Opioids?" University of Utah Health (February 20, 2017). https://healthcare.utah.edu/publicaffairs/news/2017/02/opioid-alternative.php

SERIES GLOSSARY OF KEY TERMS

abstinence—to refrain from alcohol or drug use.

analgesic—any member of a class of drugs used to achieve analgesia, or relief from pain.

antagonist—a substance that counteracts the effects of another drug, by interacting with receptors in the brain to prevent drugs from activating the receptor and causing physical or psychological effects.

cardiovascular system—the system consisting of the heart and blood vessels. It delivers nutrients and oxygen to all cells in the body.

central nervous system—the system consisting of the nerves in the brain and spinal cord. These are greatly affected by opiates and opioids.

cerebellum—a part of the brain that helps regulate posture, balance, and coordination. It is also involved in the processes of emotion, motivation, memory, and thought.

chronic condition—a medical condition that persists for a long time (at least three months or more).

craving—an intense desire for a substance, also called "psychological dependence."

dependence—a situation that occurs when opiates or opioids are used so much that the user's body adapts to the drug and only functions normally when the drug is present. When the user attempts to stop using the drug, a physiologic reaction known as withdrawal syndrome occurs.

detoxification—medical treatment of a drug addict or alcoholic, intended to rid the patient's bloodstream of the psychoactive substance. The addict is usually required to abstain from the drug or alcohol. Also known as "detox," or "managed withdrawal."

dopamine—a brain chemical, classified as a neurotransmitter, found in regions of the brain that regulate movement, emotion, motivation, and reinforcement of rewarding behavior. Dopamine release in reward areas of the brain is caused by all drugs to which people can become addicted.

epidemic—a widespread occurrence of a disease or illness in a community at a particular time.

intravenous—drug delivery through insertion of a needle into a vein.

intranasal—drug delivery via inhalation through the nose.

naloxone—an antagonist that blocks opioid receptors in the brain, so that they are not activated by opioid drugs. Because it can reverse the problem of opiate intoxication, it is often used to treat overdoses of opioids, such as heroin, fentanyl, or painkillers like oxycodone or hydrocodone.

neuron—a unique type of cell found in the brain and throughout the body that specializes in the transmission and processing of information. Also called a "nerve cell." opiates—a drug that is derived directly from the poppy plant, such as opium, heroin, morphine, and codeine.

opioids—synthetic drugs that affect the body in a similar way as opiate drugs. The opioids include oxycodone, hydrocodone, fentanyl, and methadone.

overdose—the use of any drug in such an amount that serious physical or mental effects occur, including permanent brain damage, coma, or death. The lethal dose of a particular drug can varies depending on the strength of the drug as well as the individual who is taking it.

relapse—a return to drug use or drinking after a period of abstinence, often accompanied by a recurrence of drug dependence.

self-medication—the use of a drug to lessen the negative effects of stress, anxiety, or other mental disorders without the guidance of a health care provider. Self-medication may lead to addiction and other drug-related problems.

withdrawal—a syndrome of often painful physical and psychological symptoms that occurs when someone stops using an addictive drug, such as an opiate or opioid. Often, the drug user will begin taking the drug again to avoid withdrawal.

Colvin, Rod. *Overcoming Prescription Drug Addiction: A Guide to Coping and Understanding*. Nebraska: Addicus, 2008.

Gonzales. Sebastian. *I Will Beat Back Pain: Getting into a Winning Mindset for Recovery*. Huntington Beach, Calif.: Performance Place Sports Care, 2018.

Graves, Harrison. *Alternative Pain Relief: A Pill-Free Tool Kit* Longs, SC: Novus Energus, 2018.

Klein, Arthur, and Dava Sobel. *Backache: The Complete Guide to Relief*. London: Robinson, 2006.

Meier, Barry. *Pain Killer: A "Wonder" Drug's Trail of Addiction and Death*. New York: Rodale, 2003.

Pinsky, Drew, et al. *When Painkillers Become Dangerous: What Everyone Needs to Know About OxyContin and Other Prescription Drugs*. Minnesota: Hazelden, 2004.

Quinones, Sam. *Dreamland: The True Tale of America's Opiate Epidemic*. New York: Bloomsbury, 2015.

Stolberg, Victor B. *Painkillers: History, Science, and Issues*. California: ABC-CLIO, 2016.

Taylor, Donald R. *Managing Patients with Chronic Pain and Opioid Addiction*. New York: Springer, 2015.

Ticks, Heather. *Holistic Pain Relief: Dr. Tick's Breakthrough Strategies to Manage and Eliminate Pain*. Novato, Calif: New World Library, 2013.

INTERNET RESOURCES

http://www.painmed.org
The American Academy of Pain Medicine's website provides current and relevant information on pain medicine, including clinical reference resources and the latest news on pain research.

https://www.webmd.com/pain-management/features/alternative-treatments
An informative article on alternative treatments for chronic pain from WebMD.

http://paindatabase.nih.gov
The Interagency Pain Research Portfolio database enables searches of over 1,200 research projects through a multitiered system. Topics are organized into themes, such as pain mechanisms, overlapping conditions, disparities, risk factors, and training and education.

https://www.healthline.com/health/pain-relief/surprising-natural-pain-killers
This article from HealthLine provides information on natural pain killers, including willow bark and numeric.

http://www.cdc.gov/az/p.html
The Centers for Disease Control and Prevention website contains an A-Z index that offers comprehensive information on health topics, including painkiller overdose.

https://www.everydayhealth.com/pain-management/photos/8-alternative-treatments-for-pain-management.aspx
Everyday Health provides information on alternative treatments for pain management at this site.

http://www.ccsa.ca/
This website delivers a wide range of publications on substance abuse in Canada. Subjects relate to prescription drugs, alcohol, youths, treatment, impaired driving, prevention, and standards—among others.

http://www.samhsa.gov/
A vast amount of research related to opioids and other substances can be performed on the Substance Abuse and Mental Health Services Administration website. The website also provides resources on national strategies and initiatives, state and local initiatives, and training and education.

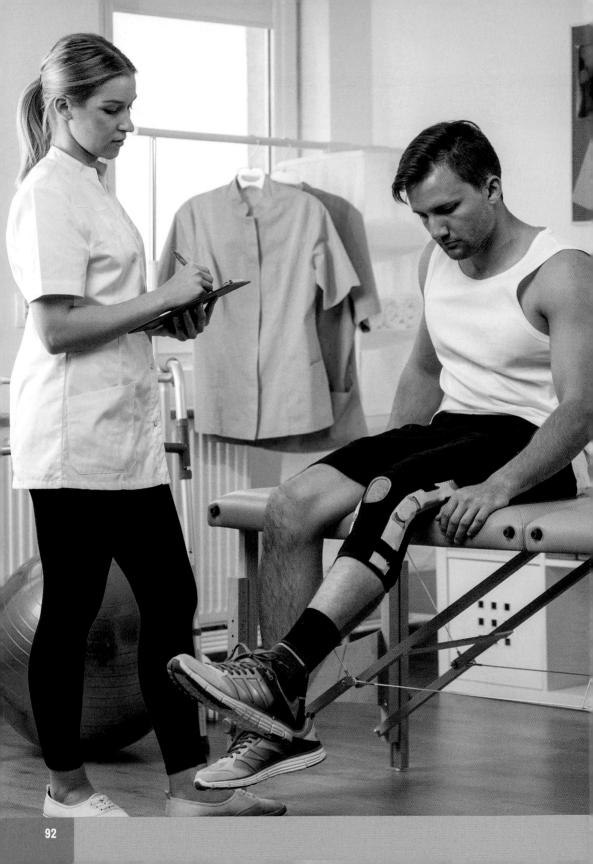

INDEX

AUTHOR'S BIOGRAPHY

Ben Baker is a newspaper publisher in South Georgia. As a newspaper reporter, he has written about the opioid epidemic and how it ravages small communities. As a journalist he has contributed to some of the nation's major daily newspapers, the Associated Press, Thomson-Reuters, and a number of magazines. This is his fifteenth book.

CREDITS